The Cancer Odyssey

The Cancer Odyssey

Discovering Truth and Inspiration
on the Way to Wellness

Margaret Brennan Bermel, MBA

To order additional copies of this book, contact:
Xlibris Corporation
1-888-795-4274
www.Xlibris.com
Orders@Xlibris.com
91921

Contents

"Re-examine all you have been told . . . dismiss that which insults your soul."

—*Walt Whitman*

Dedication

I am grateful for the miracle of my health. It is my purpose in life to awaken others to the fraud of chemotherapy. My intent is to sound the alarm: everything you have been led to believe about 'chemo' is a lie. We have to get to the tipping point where people realize, in our collective consciousness, that it is chemotherapy that is "experimental" and "controversial", not the alternative treatments. The alternatives are actually beneficial and effective. We, as a society, have been brainwashed into accepting the "standard of care"; we need to start questioning the oncological profession in order to discover the truth. Surviving cancer depends upon it.

I thank my family and friends who encouraged me to get the truth out, and my recovery "team" who helped my healing process. The articles I found on various websites exposed the truth and shaped my decisions, and were the inspiration for the vignettes that follow. The articles cited contain critical information that may help people faced with the challenge of cancer make an informed decision. These vignettes weave the story of one person; this is a very personal glimpse into my life. There are millions of us who have experienced a "cancer scare." The choices made when faced with this challenge are critical to survival. My choices shaped my life and death decision. Your choices will shape yours.

I dedicate this book to my husband, Thomas Bermel, who helped to save my life.

"Grow old along with me! The best is yet to be . . ."—*Robert Browning*

~~~

I

Preface

For the first two months after surgery, I was frozen in fear, unable to move beyond that moment in time when the doctor delivered what seemed to be my death sentence—"it was malignant." Everything in my psyche recoiled against the doctor's recommendation for "precautionary" chemotherapy, but I didn't know why. I had no hard data, no facts to support my gut feeling. So I began my odyssey into the labyrinth of the cancer industry. I was searching for a way out of cancer that did not include chemotherapy. My husband showed me an article in a Life Extension magazine, "Suzanne Somers Exposes the Cancer Establishment," which raised the question "How many cancer victims are dying needlessly?"[1] I read Somers's book *Knockout: Interview with Doctors Who Are Curing Cancer.*[2] My gut feeling was validated; there *are* alternatives to chemo. I was now on my way to wellness through truth and inspiration. I spent my recovery time surrounded by my laptop, books, and DVDs, researching chemotherapy and alternatives to chemotherapy. This is the story of my journey, and the truths and inspirations I found along the way. The e-mails to my brother Mick and others during this period were very personal sign posts along the way and are included in this preface to chronicle my thought progression: from fear and indecision to that "aha" moment—the moment of truth and inspiration.

When I started documenting my discoveries, it was with the intent to let others in my situation know that chemotherapy hurts more often than it helps. I had to find my own way back to health, in a natural, non-toxic way, and I wanted to share what I learned with others. Something happened during my journey: I moved from shock, to mistrust, to cynicism, to anger, to outrage. But then like the phoenix, I started moving from the ashes toward the light: to discovery, to truth, to inspiration. I experienced a rebirth. I discovered a very strong appreciation for my day-to-day life, and it occurred to me that a commitment to life is the key to wellness. The stories in this book reflect the complexity of the human being: we are thinking, analytical beings, yet we are also intuitive, feeling beings. The stories move from thoughts to feelings, from discovering truths about treatment choices, to finding inspiration in life. This is not a novel or a research book where one would expect chapters to unfold orderly and sequentially. This is a self-help book for the cancer patient, and it unfolds as my odyssey unfolded, in no particular order or sequence. No one in mainstream medicine can help cancer patients restore their health in a non-toxic way, and no one in alternative medicine is allowed by the FDA to claim that they can help cancer patients restore their health. The cancer patient has to take control of their own health and find their own way to restore it. This is a book of discovery, organized by a common thread that pulls all these short stories together: the common thread is truth or inspiration, or sometimes both. These thoughts and feelings go against the grain of popular, mainstream thought and opinion. All discoveries start with a departure from established thought. This book requires the reader to suspend everything that you have ever been led to believe about cancer and cancer treatments. With an open mind, you too will discover that truth and inspiration are the way to wellness. With the help of this book, you will discover your own way to wellness.

On October 26, 2009, I underwent major surgery and was diagnosed with stage 1a ovarian cancer. Although the encapsulated growths were removed, four (4) oncologists recommended "precautionary" chemotherapy treatment because the type of cancer (clear cell carcinoma) was "aggressive," and *that* is the "standard of care."

Any reference made to the medical profession in this book is to the oncological branch of medicine. Western medicine provides excellent treatment for crisis medicine: heart attacks, bullet wounds, broken legs, etc., but has been misdirected in the treatment and management of the disease called "cancer."

These personal e-mails and vignettes are organized in chronological fashion and tell my story of "discovering truth and inspiration on the way to wellness."

~~~

—Original Message—

From:	mbermel
Date:	Tuesday, November 10, 2009, 4:08 p.m.
Subject:	Hi
To:	mick

Hi Mick, I am researching alternatives to chemo. I'm not crazy about the idea of putting toxic chemicals into my body that will also kill healthy cells and weaken the immune system. Any suggestions are appreciated. I made an appointment with a nutritionist, and an endocrinologist. I am checking out naturopaths. I also contacted a cancer center in Pennsylvania, they have alternative treatment modalities to strengthen the immune system. There are websites that are anti-chemo, there is a lot of information to gather and process, and then decide what to do. A friend who is a DO (Doctor of Osteopathy) said that a "recommendation" is just that, a recommendation, but it is ultimately my decision. He suggested getting a second opinion on the chemo. The thing is, that is the standard protocol, so any oncologist will give the same standard response. There is not too much thinking 'outside the box' in that field. As you can see, I am struggling with this. ~ Margaret

The more I read, the more I started to suspect that something was amiss. Then I stumbled upon a website called "cancertutor.com."[3]

—Original Message—

From: mbermel
Date: Saturday, December 19, 2009, 2:16 p.m.
Subject: check this out.
To: mick

Check this out: "The War Between Orthodox Medicine and Alternative Medicine" on cancertutor.com. Chapter 2, "The Foundation of the War in Medicine" discusses why research into cancer cures has not progressed: the reason is essentially the profit motives of the pharmaceutical industry, the chemical industry and the petroleum industry. The cancer industry is profitable: surgery, chemotherapy, radiation are money-makers for everyone who touches this industry. That includes the pharmaceutical companies, advertising agencies, media, hospitals, manufacturers of medical equipment, and even the fund-raising charities. Because of the huge profit margin for anyone who touches this business, there is no motive to do anything differently; this is the reason that there is no progress in the "war against cancer." The article states that advances in cancer treatments have been suppressed for the past 80+ years by cancer industry leaders. The article goes on to discuss the Ralph Moss story, who was fired by Memorial Sloan-Kettering (S-K) Cancer Center for releasing the suppressed study of Dr. Kanematsu Sugiura, who had repeatedly gotten positive results in shrinking tumors in mice studies by using laetrile (Vitamin B-17). Moss found that S-K's Board of Directors included leaders of petrochemical and pharmaceutical companies, and that members of the Board also served on the Boards of media corporations. S-K's investment portfolio included holdings in these same pharmaceutical companies. ~ Margaret

This is not an altruistic industry, trying to save people's lives. This is, pure and simple, a business.

And then a very innocent chain e-mail from a friend crystallized my thoughts, and triggered the torrent of words that created the collection of vignettes that follow. The fear was gone.

—Original Message—

To: mbermel
From: laura
Date: Sunday, December 20, 2009, 1:05 p.m.
Subject: A small request. Just one line

THIS IS PRETTY NEAT. 93% won't forward. Small request. Just one line.

    Dear God, I pray for the cure of cancer. Amen.
    93% WON'T FORWARD THIS, WILL YOU?

~~~

The hair on the back of my neck stood up. That e-mail mobilized me. There already *are* cures for cancer, and people need to know this. All the research coalesced in my mind. I was beginning to find my way out of the cancer labyrinth. My response . . .

—Original Message—

From: mbermel
Date: Sunday, December 20, 2009, 1:51 p.m.
Subject: Re: A small request. Just one line
To: laura

Hi Laura,

I spent yesterday reading an on-line book on cancertutor.com (The War between Orthodox Medicine and Alternative Medicine).

There are many alternative "cures" for cancer, but they are not based on chemotherapy or radiation treatments, so the FDA and Big Pharma (the pharmaceutical companies) suppress them. The general public does not have the information to make an informed decision. Chemotherapy is the biggest scam in history, and it has to be revealed for what it is.

One of the best sites for an overall view is cancertutor.com. This entire odyssey has been a revelation: the medical oncology profession is driven by the pharmaceutical industry and the American public has been brainwashed by both. The more I read, the more I thank God that I trusted my gut on this and didn't just go along with "medical advice." I am convinced that if I had, I would not live long enough to collect Social Security. It just does not work, it is pure and utter BS. The alternative approaches that DO work are suppressed by the collusion of Big Pharma, FDA, AMA, and Congress.

The public must know this. I lost one of my best friends 4 years ago to chemotherapy (looking back, I realize it was NOT to cancer, but to chemo). These avoidable deaths of our family and friends—not just mine, yours also—must stop!

I don't "pray for the cure." My "prayer" is that people will be allowed to receive the information they need, and can exercise the freedom of choice so that they can regain their health, and stop accepting and believing that they must die a slow, painful death from the poisons administered by conventional oncology and pharmacy.

My hope is that someone will get the word out to the unsuspecting public. This is a travesty. The answer is in nature and natural solutions, not in the chemistry lab, where chemists produce one toxin after another, without regard to the collateral damage. And they don't even look for the cause! My husband asked all the oncologists we consulted, "What caused it?" All responded that they don't get involved in the cause, only the treatment. To which he responded, "if you don't know what caused it, how can you treat it?" Anyway, I feel that a path is being revealed to me, this may be my mission in life, but it is a huge challenge to get the word out. Peace, Margaret

And then on New Year's Day, I experienced my epiphany.

—Original Message—

From: mbermel
Date: Friday, January 1, 2010, 10:49 a.m.
Subject: A New Year
To: family and friends

*My New Year's Day thoughts . . . as I stand on the precipice of a new year,
I am grateful for the miracle of my health. A little over two months ago, after
extensive surgery, I received a diagnosis of stage 1a ovarian cancer. Today I
am healthy. The only moment that matters is this present moment. For me, this
has been a life-changing odyssey. I have been blessed with receiving this lesson
to pause and enjoy life and appreciate the love of family and friends. At the
beginning of this new year, I affirm the joy that life brings, and hope that all
who are dear to me find that same joy (and without having to experience the
pain that brought me to this level). Happy 2010.*
    Peace, Love, Happiness. Margaret

The vignettes that follow trace my way to wellness through truth and
inspiration.

<p align="center">~~~</p>

[1]   William Faloon, "So Many Needless Cancer Deaths," *Life Extension* Dec. 2009:
      7-12.
[2]   Suzanne Somers, *Knockout: Interviews with Doctors who are Curing Cancer and
      How to Prevent Getting it in the First Place* (New York: Crown Publishing Group,
      a division of Random House, Inc., 2009).
[3]   "The War between Orthodox Medicine and Alternative Medicine," 19 Dec.
      2009 <http://www.cancertutor.com>.

II

Vignettes

Friday, January 1, 2010

1. Don't Be Scared into Chemotherapy

I have firsthand experience with the health care system. For the past nine (9) weeks, I have been researching and meeting with conventional oncologists, and it is my opinion that cancer is a multi-billion dollar business. Period. Chemotherapy (chemo) is the biggest fraud ever perpetrated upon the American public, and we are all paying for it. The pharmaceutical companies are the big winners. Americans are being led to slaughter like sheep; it is not cancer that kills, it is the "chemo" that kills. If this were exposed for the fraud that it is, many businesses would lose a lot of money, so the fraud must continue. Some of the truths that I have discovered: 1) The statistics are skewed: people who decline chemo treatment are *not* included in the stats. There is *no* control group. I know five (5) people personally who declined treatment and who are healthy; they are not followed in a longitudinal study. The statistics are based solely upon people who *accept* treatment. I knew fifteen (15) people personally who had chemo and who are now dead. The Surveillance, Epidemiology, and End Results (SEER) Program of the National Cancer Institute (NCI) generates these statistics, yet the statistics do not tell the entire story. The major omission in the statistical analysis is how effective this type of treatment is compared to other types of treatments, or to no treatment at all. 2) Chemo is effective on only three (3) different types of cancers (testicular, lymphoma, and childhood leukemia), yet it is presented as treatment for *all* cancers, even though it is known to be ineffective. 3) Chemo can cause other cancers to occur. 4) Chemo can make cancer cells resistant to all chemo treatments. Cancer cells fight to survive chemo by adapting and mutating, and then they divide even faster, and develop a resistance to chemo. 5) The basic premise of chemo needs to be questioned: the shotgun approach with collateral damage to organs and immune system is *not* acceptable. 6) Oncologists routinely use scare tactics about length of life to induce people to agree to accept toxic chemo, when there is no proof that the treatment will benefit the individual patient. 7) There are other wellness plans that would benefit people, but these plans are blocked by the Food and Drug Administration (FDA), the American Medical Association (AMA), and the pharmaceutical industry (Big Pharma). 8) It is more beneficial to strengthen the immune system than to weaken it. Chemo weakens it. 9) Oncologists are legally required to offer chemo as the "standard of care," and if the patient declines, the declination is documented to limit medical liability. There are many websites and documentaries that document these truths in detail.[1,2]

This is the crux of the health care problem. This is where the money goes. Insurance companies cover only the conventional therapies, because people have been brainwashed into believing that chemo is the only option when faced with a cancer diagnosis. Unless people start to question the basic premise of chemo, it will remain the knee-jerk reaction to cancer. The unnecessary deaths of almost 600,000 Americans every year from chemotherapy must be stopped. According to the American Cancer Society, there are 569,490 Americans who are expected to die of cancer in 2010.[3] It is not conclusive, in my mind, that people die of *cancer*. I believe that it is more likely that people are dying of the "cure"—*chemotherapy*.

During my recovery time from surgery, I researched treatment options, and I have discovered how ineffective this "treatment" really is. My husband and I consulted with several oncologists, one of whom worked at MD Anderson Cancer Center for many years, followed by a brief stint with a pharmaceutical company before returning to another "cancer center." This doctor responded truthfully to all our questions, and in effect confirmed that there *are* no studies which would indicate that chemo would benefit *me*, that chemo can cause other cancers, that chemo could result in cancer cells mutating and becoming resistant to all chemo drugs, and finally, that if I declined treatment, he would not see me again. I would not be offered any type of alternative treatment. I would not be monitored to track my health status. I would not be included in a control group. I would not be studied longitudinally to track my progress using an alternative approach to chemo. The treatment was chemo: take it or leave it.

There is no comparison between people who opt for chemo treatments and people who opt for alternative treatments. When the oncologist presents to the patient the "statistics" which are provided by the pharmaceutical companies, the patient should be aware that these statistics are skewed, and therefore meaningless. The statistics become the sales pitch to create a sense of urgency and to scare people into "treatment." The "treatment" is beneficial only to the bottom line of the cancer industry.

It has been a revelation to me that the oncological profession is driven by the pharmaceutical industry, which is driven by the profit motive. The American public has been brainwashed. This is the truth. Recognize it.

---

[1]   "The War between Orthodox Medicine and Alternative Medicine," 19 Dec. 2009 <http://www.cancertutor.com>.

[2]   *Healing Cancer from the Inside Out*, dir. Mike Anderson, DVD, 2008).

[3]   "Cancer Facts & Figures 2010," American Cancer Society, 2010, <http://www. cancer.org/Research/CancerFactsFigures/CancerFactsFigures/cancer-facts-and-figures-2010>.

Saturday, January 2, 2010

2. "A rose is a rose is a rose . . ."

Chemotherapy is a toxic poison. It is not a cure for cancer. A "cure" for cancer, as defined by the oncological establishment, occurs when the length of life from diagnosis passes the five (5) year mark.[1] If the patient is still alive, the patient is deemed to be cured, regardless of the physical condition of the patient. The patient may actually die after five (5) years and one (1) day, but that is irrelevant; the patient is counted in the statistics as a success of chemotherapy.

Think about this objectively: if you were given a medication for a disease that caused your hair to fall out, wouldn't you refuse to take that medication? Of course you would. However, the American public has been brainwashed into accepting complete hair loss as collateral damage. But this is *not* acceptable. If there is a visible manifestation such as hair loss, just imagine, really imagine, the havoc that chemotherapy is wreaking *within* the body.

Chemotherapy is experimental therapy that is embraced as the mainstream medical solution to cancer. It is not the solution. It was developed from the mustard gas used in the World Wars.[2,3] It is not effective against most cancers; 97% of the time, it just does not work.[4]

If it worked, if people were actually cured by this toxin, then hair loss would be an acceptable side effect, as would be immune system destruction, and healthy cell and organ destruction, and all the other numerous side effects. This would all be acceptable, if only this treatment actually worked! But it does not work. I have had two (2) oncologists hand me the drug information pamphlets (as they are legally required to do), and then both said to me "but don't read them too closely," with one of the oncologists adding, "they make the side effects sound really bad." The truth is—the side effects *are* really bad.

The media propaganda, which is fed by the pharmaceutical companies, leads the public to believe that "the cure is right around the corner," and that there have been advances in chemotherapy in the past twenty (20) years with increased survival rates. This is simply untrue. Chemotherapy twenty (20) years ago was horrible; today it is just terrible, and just as ineffective.

It is important to differentiate the cause of death: is it the cancer that is the cause of death, or is it the chemo? When you see someone who visibly manifests the hair loss side effect of chemotherapy, it is important to acknowledge that this is a *chemo* patient. Cancer does not cause hair loss. Chemo causes hair loss. This person is not being treated properly for cancer; this person is being administered a toxic poison.

People should not accept this "treatment" without researching and questioning it. We have all been brainwashed by the propaganda generated by the oncological business, pharmaceutical companies, media (which benefits from advertising revenue from Big Pharma), and the FDA. All are complicit; all are in tacit collusion to perpetrate this fraud. People research vacation choices, real estate choices, education choices, and career choices. People must start researching their health choices; it is a matter of life or death.

I have lost loved ones to this "treatment," a regimen which should be considered experimental and controversial, and I came very close to becoming a statistic myself.

"A rose is a rose is a rose . . ." (Gertrude Stein, 1913). "Chemo is a poison is a poison is a poison" (Charlotte Gerson). [5] People deserve to know the truth. Without the truth, there is no way to wellness.

---

[1] *Healing Cancer from the Inside Out*, dir. Mike Anderson, DVD, 2008).

[2] Wikipedia, <http://en.Wikipedia.org/wiki/chemotherapy>.

[3] Dr. Laurence Magne, "Chemotherapy: Does it Really Cause Cancer?," <http://searchwarp.com/ swa78335.htm>.

[4] Anderson.

[5] Anderson.

Sunday, January 3, 2010

3. "The truth shall set us free"

I am grateful for the miracle of my health. It is my purpose in life to awaken others to the myth of chemo. The intent of these vignettes is to sound the alarm: everything you are led to believe about chemo is a lie.

I affirm that I am healthy. Any thoughts about cancer or chemotherapy are not intended to attract any negative energy back to me. The thoughts are transformed into positive energy which is intended to help others who need this information at this time. Those people will be led to these vignettes to help them find their truth. I found the truth by spending my recovery time from extensive surgery—six (6) weeks at home—on my laptop searching and researching the truth. I am grateful that I discovered the truth before I signed up for "death by chemo." Believe this: chemotherapy is a slow, painful death in many, many cases. Do your due diligence and make sure you know what you are getting into.

I am healthy and I affirm the positive power of transitioning a negative into a positive. These vignettes are my personal opinion, based on my research, and are a means of sharing the personal experiences of my unintentional foray into the cancer industry. These vignettes are intended to be thought-provoking only. You must find your own truth: "the truth shall set us free."

Sunday, January 3, 2010

4. We Can't Bring Back Those We Lost to Chemo

Everyone knows someone who they think died from cancer. I have lost people I love dearly, I thought, to cancer. I *thought* that they died from cancer; now I know that the actual cause of death was chemotherapy. Their deaths push me to help get the truth out. I wish that I knew then what I know now. Would they still be here? That is unknown. Maybe. Maybe not. We can't go back in time. We can't bring back those we lost. We can only look forward. It is only a matter of time before someone you know hears the words that I heard when the surgeon leaned over me in the recovery room and said "it was malignant . . ." Our environment is toxic, our stress levels are high, and it seems to be a question of not "if" but "when" that diagnosis will be made. Be prepared to "just say no to chemo." Be aware that the cancer industry is based on the ability to create fear, making it very easy to manipulate people into chemotherapy. Let's try to save everyone that we can in the future.

My close brush with chemotherapy pushes me to help get the truth out. I am grateful to my husband. The week after surgery, the oncologist recommended "precautionary chemotherapy." My husband asked me what I was going to do. I replied, "Of course I'll do it, I will do everything I can to beat this." This was the fearful, knee-jerk reaction that the cancer industry counts on. I had been subliminally brainwashed over the years, and I was ready to sign on the dotted line. What the cancer industry doesn't count on is a husband who says what my husband said: "Let's not be too hasty, let's research this." I am grateful every day that he had the wisdom to speak those words.

The body has a tremendous ability to heal. According to Charlotte Gerson, daughter of Dr. Max Gerson, "You cannot heal with poison."[1] Give the body what it needs to heal. Trust. You will heal. "Just say no to chemo."

---

[1]   *Healing Cancer from the Inside Out*, dir. Mike Anderson, DVD, 2008).

Monday, January 4, 2010

5. "The emperor wears no clothes"

How many times have you heard that someone was diagnosed with cancer and died three (3) months later? Question: did they have chemotherapy? If yes, what was the "real" cause of death—chemo or cancer? I put my money on chemo. And so do the pharmaceutical companies. Even when patients are terminal with no hope of recovery, the poison continues to be administered. This is shameless corporate greed and nothing more. Remember the lesson of how Wall Street caused the implosion of the economy; the pharmaceutical industry—"Big Pharma"—is just as greedy, corrupt, and ruthless as their counterparts in the investment and banking industry have been exposed to be.

If you signed up for chemo and you cannot cite the research study which proves that chemo will cure *your* disease, then you have no "evidence-based" data to support your decision. I am not talking about regurgitating the skewed stats that your oncologist spewed out about your five (5) year survival rate and the percentage probability that your disease will recur. I am talking "show me the money"—what is your *source*? If you cannot cite a source, then you have been deceived. Incidentally, the stats that the oncologist spews forth are sourced by the drug salesman from Big Pharma, and are presented in relative numbers, not absolute numbers. According to Disraeli, and later Mark Twain, there are three types of lies: " . . . lies, damn lies, and statistics." These misleading statistics paint the picture the cancer industry wants to paint, and the cancer patient is painted into a corner, cowering in fear. You will agree to anything to save your life. You *think* that you are saving your life, but you have in actuality just signed your own death certificate.

The only benefit of chemotherapy is to the bottom line of the cancer industry. Don't help the cancer industry perpetuate the myth. Educate yourself. Knowledge is power.

People accept chemotherapy unquestioningly, afraid of being ridiculed or of not going along with conventional thinking. Dr. Ulrich Abel, a German epidemiologist, conducted an extensive study in the 1980s and declared chemotherapy to be a "scientific wasteland," and stated that "chemotherapy can rarely improve the quality of life." His study found an effectiveness rate of 3%, and stated that "at least 80 percent of chemotherapy administered throughout the world is worthless, and is akin to the 'emperor's new clothes'—neither doctor nor patient is willing to give up on chemotherapy even though there is no scientific evidence that it works."[1]

Well-intentioned family and friends will become very upset when they learn of your decision to decline chemotherapy. They will try to convince you to reconsider, but they will be hard-pressed to explain *why*. I have had many people comment that I am very brave to go against medical advice; it is actually a matter of being resolute, not brave, and being able to stand your ground against the pressure of family and friends. In my opinion, people who accept chemotherapy are the brave ones. They are unknowingly walking into the hell called chemotherapy. I was scared to death of chemotherapy; I wanted no part of it. I made my decision based on truth, and I have been resolute in standing by the decision. My bravery lies in my determination to let others know what I have discovered.

Be brave enough to call out, "The emperor wears no clothes." This is truth; do not be afraid to expose it.

---

[1]   Dr. George J Georgiou, Ph.D.,ND.,D.Sc (AM), "Are We Treating Cancer but Killing the Patient?", <<http://www.rawfoodinfo.com/articles/art_arewe treating cancerbutkillingpatient. htm>>.

Monday, January 4, 2010

6. An Unholy Alliance

An unholy alliance has developed over the last century that created the tangled web called the cancer industry. The common strand linking all the players in this web is the pharmaceutical industry, "Big Pharma." Until the strand connecting Big Pharma with the medical schools is severed, and the medical establishment can independently and objectively determine *if* pharmaceuticals are the correct course of action in the treatment of a disease, the American public will continue to believe in the deception that drugs are the quick fix to every medical ailment. The training of doctors to rely on pharmaceuticals starts in medical school, and then the doctors emerge to train the patients. Doctors are *not* trained on natural supplements or vitamins; their knowledge in this field is actually inferior to that of the average person's knowledge about natural supplements or vitamins. Part of the medical training is to condescendingly dismiss vitamins and supplements as quackery.

Cancer Centers and Big Business:

"The world's oldest and largest private cancer center, Memorial Sloan-Kettering Cancer Center (MSKCC) . . . founded in 1884 as the New York Cancer Hospital by a group that included John J. Astor and his wife, Charlotte, the original building on the Upper West Side of Manhattan began its move to its present location on York Avenue in 1936 when John D. Rockefeller, Jr. donated the land upon which, in 1939, Memorial Hospital was constructed. Between 1970 and 1973, a new Memorial Hospital was constructed and this building stands on the site today.

In the 1940s, two former General Motors executives, Alfred P. Sloan and Charles F. Kettering, joined forces to establish the Sloan-Kettering Institute (SKI). SKI has since become one of the nation's premier biomedical research institutions."[1]

Big Pharma and the FDA:

"The Dirty Little Secret between the FDA and the Drug Industry"[2] describes the relationship between the FDA and the very industry that it is charged with overseeing. Very often, FDA officials find a soft landing spot in a pharmaceutical company after retirement from the FDA. Big Pharma, in a close alliance with the FDA, has developed a virtual monopoly on the cancer business. It is a business. Any alternative natural treatments which are beneficial to people are suppressed by the FDA. Only chemical substances can be patented; natural substances cannot be patented. The bottom line profits from the sale of chemotherapy drugs; the cost of research and development, and of course, the profit margin, is factored into the cost of the drugs. Natural substances do not generate the billions of dollars that chemical substances do. Natural substances are viewed as a threat because they are comparatively cheap, they actually work, and are consequently and systematically discredited by the FDA.

Big Pharma and the American Cancer Society and the National Cancer Institute

The American Cancer Society and the National Cancer Institute are embedded institutions with the goal of self-perpetuation. The interest is in getting the public to believe that the "cure is right around the corner," thereby getting the public to make donations, much of which goes to the pharmaceutical companies to continue research and development (R&D) for newer and more profitable chemical solutions.

Big Pharma and the Media:

Can you watch TV without being bombarded by advertisements for drugs?

These ads target the baby boomers, subliminally infiltrating the conscious and subconscious minds, planting the seed of disease. Hit the mute button. We are healthy and do not need Big Pharma's wares.

Big Pharma and the Medical Profession:

Oncologists receive incentives from every patient they sign up for chemo.

They are legitimized drug dealers. Don't deal with them. Oncologists receive what is referred to as the "chemotherapy concession," which means that they can pocket the difference between their cost and the amount of insurance reimbursement. This "concession" may influence a patient's treatment. A study published in *Health Affairs* revealed that "financial reimbursement has a direct effect on which chemotherapy drugs are prescribed to patients."[3] Doctors typically buy drugs and benefit not only from the "concession," but also receive rebates based on the amount they have purchased. Although federal laws prohibit drug companies from paying doctors for prescribing pills, there is no regulation that bans payment for intravenous drugs.[4]

Big Pharma and Medical Schools:

Pharmaceutical companies provide funding to medical schools and influence the curriculum in terms of the "standard of care" for cancer treatment.[5,6] Until the "arms-length" relationship between the medical schools and the pharmaceutical industry can be re-established, the role of doctors is compromised; they have become prescribers of drugs, not the omniscient healers of disease that the American public imagines they are.

Any alternative treatment practitioners are shut down by the FDA; it is literally against the law to find a real cure that does not involve toxic chemicals. The unholy alliance of Big Pharma, the FDA, the fund-raising societies, the government research agencies, the medical institutions, and big business: did the American public *ever* have a chance? This group is *not* trying to save mankind from disease. This is *not* altruism; this is greed. Pure and simple.

With a diagnosis of cancer, the immediate knee-jerk reaction is to go into the medical institution established by big business and sign up for chemo. And when you walk into a treatment facility, you are a potential $100,000 sale. Minimum. For that money, will you walk out healthy? Will you walk out alive? What does that $100,000 buy you? Certainly, no guarantees. This is not about your health. It is always about the money. The profit motive is at work here.

"In times of universal deceit, telling the truth will be a revolutionary act." (George Orwell). Do not believe what you are told without first questioning and researching. These are the worst kind of drug dealers. This is *your* life. Take it into your own hands. This is truth.

---

[1]   "Memorial Sloan-Kettering Cancer Center," <http://wwwmskcc.org/ mskcc/ html/511.cfm>.

[2]   Chris Gupta, "The Dirty Little Secret between the FDA and the Drug Industry", <http://www.communicationagents.com/chris/2004/08/26/the_dirty_ little_ secret_between_the_fda_and_drug_industry.htm>

[3]   "Oncologists profit on chemotherapy drugs they prescribe to cancer patients," Apr. 2006, <http://www.mesothel.com/asbestos-cancer/mesothelioma/ chemotherapy/alimta/alimta_profit.htm>.

[4]   "The Danger in Drug Kickbacks," The New York Times, 14 May 2007, <http:// www.nytimes.com/2007/05/14/opinion/14mon1.html?_r=1>.

[5]   Duff Wilson, "Harvard Teaching Hospitals Cap Outside Pay," The New York Times, 2 Jan. 2010, <http://www.nytimes.com/2010/01/03/health/ research/03hospital.html?emc=eta1>.

[6]   Duff Wilson, "Harvard Medical School in Ethics Quandary," The New York Times, 2 Mar. 2009, <http://www.nytimes.com/2009/03/03/business/ 03medschool.html?emc=eta1%3C/div>.

Monday, January 4, 2010

7. Boycott Chemo

Anyone who was either at Woodstock or regretted missing Woodstock was a self-proclaimed "hippie." In subsequent years, that term came to carry some negative connotations, as many hippies ultimately self-destructed, getting permanently lost while trying to find themselves. At some point, most hippies realized that they had to get their acts together and get a real job; then we became "baby boomers." However, as a group, hippies actually achieved the impossible: we protested the Vietnam War, we called upon Nixon to resign, we even boycotted lettuce to protest the poor working conditions of migrant workers. "The fight is never about grapes or lettuce. It is always about people." (Cesar Chavez).

Although I missed Woodstock, and regretted missing it (I turned sixteen that weekend and my mother would not allow me to go), I do recall a scene from the movie *Woodstock*, where an announcement was made warning people about some drugs that were circulating. The announcement was, "that's some bad shit man, stay away from it!"

Chemotherapy is "some bad shit man," stay away from it! "Now is the time for all [old hippies] to come to the aid of [each other]." Stop this travesty. It is a real paradigm shift to understand that chemo is *not* the only way to go. You must wrap your mind around it. There is a book called *Chemotherapy Heals Cancer and the World is Flat* by Lothar Hirneise.[1] The title says it all. There are safer, non-toxic solutions. Find them. The sheer number of baby boomers can move this protest to the tipping point where we all refuse to do the "bad shit" being pushed by Big Pharma. Stand up. Question. Read. Research. Demand answers.

The hippie/baby boomer generation was about being "anti-establishment." The struggle was against the oppression of the old guard. We fought that battle and made breakthrough strides which created a freer society. It is time to once again struggle against the old guard of the cancer industry, time once again to become "anti-establishment."

"The fight . . . is about people." Boycott chemo. Seek the truth. Find your inspiration.

---

[1] "Lothar Hirneise's Book *Chemotherapy Heals Cancer and the World is Flat*: Extract/Table of Contents," <http://www.healingcancernaturally.com/ hirneise-chemotherapy-cures.html>.

Tuesday, January 5, 2010

8.   Primum Non Nocere

"Primum non nocere is a Latin phrase that means 'First, do no harm.' Nonmaleficence, which derives from the maxim, is one of the principal precepts of medical ethics that all medical students are taught in medical school, and is a fundamental principle for emergency medical services around the world. Another way to state it is that 'given an existing problem, it may be better to do nothing than to do something that risks causing more harm than good.' It reminds the physician and other health care providers that they must consider the possible harm that any intervention might do. It is invoked when debating the use of an intervention that carries an obvious risk of harm, but a less certain chance of benefit. Since at least 1860, the phrase has been, for physicians, a hallowed expression of hope, intention, humility, and recognition that human acts with good intentions may have unwanted consequences. A closely related phrase is 'Sometimes the cure is worse than the ill.' The origin of the phrase is uncertain. The Hippocratic Oath includes the promise 'to abstain from doing harm' but not the precise phrase. Perhaps the closest approximation in the Hippocratic Corpus is in Epidemics: 'The physician must . . . have two special objects in view with regard to disease, namely, to do good or to do no harm.'"[1]

Doctors who administer chemotherapy, in most cases, are *first, doing harm.*

This is a violation of their own Hippocratic Oath. These are intelligent people; they have to realize that they are harming the immune system, harming healthy cells, harming healthy organs, harming the nervous system. Chemo is a very harmful treatment, often causing more harm than good. First, do no harm? Chemo harms and should be abandoned as a treatment option.

The oncology profession must be reminded: *"Primum non nocere."* This is truth. *Veritas.*

---

[1]   Wikipedia, <http://en.wikipedia.org>.

Tuesday, January 5, 2010

9.   The Path to Excellent Health

I can only relay my story, and what I have found to work for *my* health crisis. If chemo is *not* the answer, what is? If chemo doesn't work, what does?

Essentially, the path to excellent health is through good nutrition, supplementation, exercise and body work, positive thinking, spiritual centering, mind-body connection, and *joie de vivre*.

That sounds very trite and too simple. Shouldn't we have to really suffer to beat this thing? *No.*

When a cancer diagnosis is dropped on you, it is one of the biggest shocks of your life. It is totally unexpected; it comes out of left field. You are blindsided. If I hadn't been lying on a gurney, I would have fallen to the floor. At that very instant, your entire being makes the decision: live or die. I made the decision to live.

Getting through the physical discomfort of the recuperation process was the initial challenge. Compounding the physical issues is dealing with the fear of death. It is a huge challenge to bring this under control. The oncologists plant the seed of fear in your mind. What if they are right? What if I am wrong? You are plagued by doubts that must be dispelled for this to work.

Put together a support team of health care practitioners. This is what works:

Unconventional medical assistance

Find a doctor who thinks outside the box. The clue is in the name of the medical facility. Avoid centers with the word "cancer" in the name: they focus on the disease. Find a center with the word "wellness" in the name: they focus on health. You need to find a medical professional who will allow you to trust your decision not to accept conventional chemotherapy. I found a respected doctor, and he gave me his medical blessing: *it is OK* to reject the conventional standard of care. You *can* go "AMA" (against medical advice). This is *your* decision. And you *will* live. His medical advice: strengthen the immune system, eat healthy foods, exercise, be happy.

Good nutrition

Cancer *loves* sugar. Give it up. Now. In all forms. Eat whole grains and vegetables. Go to the health food store for guidance. Buy books: *The*

Anti-Cancer Cookbook by Julia Greer, MD, MPH; *Beating Cancer with Nutrition* by Patrick Quillin, PhD, RD, CNS.[1,2] There are a lot of good books out there. Go to Borders and browse, or go to Amazon.com and browse. Go to your local health food store. Find an organic supermarket. Find an organic cafe that has a meal plan and will make wholesome meals for pickup. Eat all the superfoods: green tea, berries, red grapes, tomatoes, broccoli, cauliflower, garlic, onions. Sprinkle turmeric on everything. Avoid high fructose corn syrup (HFCS). Avoid artificial sweeteners and diet sodas. Don't be taken in by the marketing of these products that claim that these additives are harmless; they are not harmless. Drink filtered water. Your internal environment has to be so healthy that cancer cannot survive it. There is truth in the maxim "You are what you eat." A nutritionist at a "cancer center" told me to follow the food pyramid. Nutritionists in "cancer centers" do not think outside the box. I walked out and did not return.

Supplementation

Take antioxidants (Selenium, Vitamins C and E); Resveratrol, Probiotics, Cinnamon, Ginger, B Complex, CoQ10, Fish Oil, Vitamin D, Turmeric, Coriolus. Do not buy drug store vitamins. Go to your local health food store and talk to the proprietor. Join Life Extension.[3] Not all vitamins are created equal. The same nutritionist who told me to follow the food pyramid also told me that she did not believe in vitamins or supplements because all the vitamins that the body requires should come from food. She did not believe in Vitamin C, because it is not "evidence-based." I questioned how the body of work compiled by the Nobel Prize winner Linus Pauling could not be considered "evidence-based." The nutritionist had no answer to that. When you hear something that is not truth, if statements are made that lack credibility and integrity, get up and walk out.

Exercise and Body work

Cancer *hates* oxygen. Walking Chi Gung (Guo Lin Qi Gong) is a free video available online.[4,5] Hundreds of thousands of healthy cancer patients who practice martial art in China cannot be wrong. I started doing Chi Gung post-surgically as soon as I could walk. I also bought a Chi Gung tape to follow along with, and resumed my Chi Gung class. Chi Gung focuses on deep breathing. The key is to overcoming cancer is to oxygenate the cells. Stress-reduction body work should be enjoyed regularly. Have medical massages. Have spa massages. Acupuncture. Acupressure. Reflexology. Chiropractic. If the body is stressed, you cannot heal.

Positive thinking

Surround yourself with people who think positively. Before my surgery, a person who is a motivational speaker came into my life through golf. Ruth and I enjoyed the game, and had some conversations along the way. When she learned of my challenge, she would encourage me, by saying "have an expectancy of good," and other very positive expressions. I found this to be enormously helpful. There are a lot of very positive books, CDs, and DVDs. Listen to meditation tapes, and read and listen to Louise Hay, and Esther and Jerry Hicks.[6,7,8,9] Learn how to use affirmations; learn how to meditate. You need a very strong support group of people who love you. I am fortunate to have a spouse who has been my rock throughout this challenge. Allow your loved ones to help, and express your gratitude. Stop being a Type A personality. Now! Do not accept the concept of "remission." Remission implies that the disease will return, and that the healthy physical state is but a brief respite. Do not accept this negative thought. Believe that you are robustly healthy, and that you will continue to be robustly healthy. Do not allow your mind to wait for disease to return.

Spiritual Centering

Make your peace with your God. Find spiritual healing through organized religion or other means. Use healing crystals, magnets, holy medals, talismans. Balance your chi. Let go of the past. Forgive past wrongs. Give up the sadness and grief of losing loved ones. Let it go. You must for your own well-being. Connect with spirit. Tap into the universal life force. Find peace and tranquility.

Mind-Body Connection

Where the mind goes, the body follows. Think very positive, healing thoughts. Go to a Reiki master, a healing circle, a healing touch practitioner, a psychotherapist, a medical intuitive. Get all the help you possibly can. What *not* to do: do not join a cancer survivor support group. You do not want to talk about disease. This is the Law of Attraction at work: you attract what you focus on. If you aren't familiar with the Law of Attraction, buy the Hicks CDs.[10]

Joie de vivre

This is most important: you must start to find joy in everyday life. Smile at yourself in the mirror. Smile at your spouse. Laugh at least once an hour.

Start generating the endorphins. After receiving a death sentence, the only way to commute the sentence is to laugh your way out of it. Watch comedies, go to comedy shows, find anything to laugh at.

Raison d'être

You must find your purpose in life, your reason for being. Use your right side of the brain and create something: a beautiful garden, a painting, music, a book. Channel your inner experiences into something amazing. Letting the creative juices flow can help restore your balance in life, and can help you find your own unique reason for your very existence. We are not just here to pass the time. Find your mission in life. Do something positive every day; first for yourself, and then for others. Challenge yourself every day; push beyond the limits of the day before.

With the experience of cancer, an amazing thing happens: you become grateful for every day, for every moment of every day. It is a reawakening, a rebirth. Life is good.

And the best part of this approach to overcoming cancer is that none of these things are toxic, they don't hurt, they won't kill you, and they *will* help you discover the way to wellness through truth and inspiration. This is the path to excellent health.

1   Julia Greer, MD, MPH, *The Anti-Cancer Cookbook*, (North Branch, MN: Sunrise River Press, 2008).

2   Patrick Quillen, PhD, *Beating Cancer with Nutrition*, (Carlsbad, CA: Nutrition Times Press, Inc., 2005).

3   <http://www.lef.org>.

4   "Guolin Qi Gong-Cancer Buster. Walking Qi Gong." <http://www.qigongchinesehealth.com/walking_qigong>.

5   *Our Exclusive Guo Lin Chi Gong Video*, <http://www.healthyfoundations. com/guolin/guolin_video.html>.

6   *"Louise Hay | Author and Founder of Hay House, Inc.,"* <http://www.louisehay.com/affirmations/index.php>.

7   *Cancer: Discovering your Healing Power*, dir Louise Hay, DVD. Hay House, Inc., 2004.

8   Louise L. Hay, *You Can Heal Your Life*, New York, Hay House, Inc., 2008.

9   Esther and Jerry Hicks, *The Law of Attraction*, New York, Hay House, Inc., 2007.

10   Hicks.

Thursday, January 7, 2010

10. How Effective IS Chemotherapy?

When presented with the recommendation of chemotherapy, people assume that this is an effective medication that actually works to eliminate the disease of cancer from your body. Why else would it be recommended? Prior to all my research, if I had to guess the effectiveness of chemotherapy treatment, if asked, "what is the percentage of people who are cured by chemotherapy?" I would say, "well, I do know of some people who have had chemotherapy, and who still died anyway, so I know that it is not 100% effective, so I'll guess, it is probably around 85% effective."

WRONG, WRONG, WRONG!

In a study conducted outside the U.S., where the results could *not* be suppressed by the FDA, Dr. Ulrich Abel, a biostatistician, published a meta-analysis on survival rates of chemotherapy-treated patients. Of the cancers which can kill 80% of cancer patients (with the remaining 20% of cancer patients having non-lethal forms of skin cancer), chemotherapy alone is effective for only 3% of these patients. 3%. Let me repeat that. 3%. Wrap your mind around that number. 3%! That is abysmal. And criminal. Not even close to my 85% guess. I was off by 82%! How far off were you? I am willing to guess that you missed the mark as well, because these statistics are *not* revealed to the American public. Chemotherapy, in most cases, is *not* an effective treatment modality.[1,2,3]

The Beautiful Truth investigates the claims of Gerson Therapy, a healthy living regimen founded by Dr. Max Gerson who cured cancer and other diseases with a plant-based diet which boosts the body's immune system. Dr. Gerson was disparaged by the medical organizations in this country in the early 1920s, because he claimed that these organizations suppressed natural cancer cures. Dr. Gerson's work has been continued by his daughter Charlotte Gerson, who states, "There are laws against healing cancer. The doctor is not allowed to try anything else. He *must* use only those treatments that have already been proven to be failures. Imagine what we could do if this would be accepted. But there are laws against it. You are not allowed to heal. There is too much money to be made on drugs." Ms. Gerson states that Gerson Therapy is a cure for cancer, a statement that is supported by doctors in other countries who claim to have the medical files to prove it. Ms. Gerson further states that "the Cancer Industry has limited the choice of therapies to the worst kinds of treatments (surgery, radiation, chemotherapy), while criminalizing alternative therapies (lose medical license, jail, fines). When the cancer comes back, the doctor is not allowed to try anything other than the things that have failed, so the patient is sentenced to death, and that is criminal."[4] There are two (2) licensed Gerson Therapy treatment centers, one in Mexico and one in Hungary.[5] The treatment center in the U.S. was forced by the FDA to shut down.[6]

In a 1985 study conducted by Harvard researcher, published in Scientific American, entitled *The Treatment of Diseases and the War Against Cancer*, the researcher, John Cairns, reported on the efficacy of adjuvant therapies, such as chemotherapy. Cairns concluded that overall, "the gains [from the use of chemotherapy] have been limited. For the vast majority of cancers, which arise in older patients, the results of chemotherapy are much more controversial. Apart from the success with Hodgkin's disease, childhood leukemia and a few other cancers, it is not possible to detect any sudden change in death rates for any of the major cancers that could be credited to chemotherapy."[7]

The same study showed that chemotherapy is "somewhat effective in only 2-3% of cancer patients, primarily those with the rarest kinds of cancer (Hodgkin's disease, leukemia, testicular cancer, and choriocarcinoma).[8]

Another study published in the *New England Journal of Medicine* in 1986, entitled "Progress against Cancer?," written by Harvard researchers John C. Bailar III and Elaine M. Smith, concluded that there is "no evidence that some 35 years of intense and growing efforts to improve the treatment of cancer have had much overall effect on the most fundamental measure of clinical outcome—death. We are losing the war against cancer . . . Some thirty-five years of intense effort focused largely on improving treatment must be judged a qualified failure."[9]

There are numerous websites that report that Ronald Reagan, while President, traveled to Germany and was treated by Dr. Hans Neiper for cancer. Unconfirmed reports state that Reagan declined the American "standard of care" and survived his cancer. In 1982, he reportedly fired the entire U.S. Cancer Advisory Board, a group of conventional thinkers on cancer treatment.[10] However, the secrecy surrounding his treatment helped no one but himself. President Reagan was a potential change agent, and he could have advanced health care in the U.S. He was in a position to effect change, to change the course of the "war on cancer" by telling the truth and inspiring others. Anyone in that position has the responsibility to step up and lead others onto the right path. Reagan failed the American people; he failed to lead us down the right path.

Former Vice-President Hubert Humphrey was diagnosed with bladder cancer and submitted to conventional treatment. Before his death, he referred to chemotherapy as "bottled death."[11]

Another high profile White House figure, Tony Snow, Press Secretary in the Bush administration, adhered to the American "standard of care," and as a result died after chemotherapy, metastasis, and more chemotherapy.

There are many more anecdotal stories of people who followed traditional treatment and died, and a few stories about those who declined traditional treatment and lived. There are many celebrities, and many ordinary people, who have been diagnosed with cancer. Some survive, some die. What differentiates the surviving group from the dying group? The intervening variable, the variable that determines the life or death outcome, is chemotherapy. Celebrity status, power, indomitable spirit, will power, will to survive: these attributes are no match for chemotherapy. Chemo is a small scale "weapon of mass destruction" originating as mustard gas and injected into the body. Hello? Can anyone reasonably expect to survive this onslaught? If you *do* decide to accept chemotherapy, even after realizing that the effectiveness of chemo is more folklore than fact, then at least "know before you go." Know that you are taking a path that will not restore your health. Know that you are walking into your own private battleground.

The bottom line is that chemotherapy is an ineffective treatment choice for most cancers. It will not help you get better. It will help you get worse. You must rely on your body's capability to heal. Strengthen the immune system. Listen to your common sense. This is the way to truth; this is the way to wellness.

---

[1]   <http://www.cancertutor.com>.

[2]   *Healing Cancer from the Inside Out*, dir. Mike Anderson, DVD, 2008).

[3]   Dr. George J Georgiou, Ph.D.,ND.,D.Sc (AM), "Are we treating cancer, but killing the patient?",<http://www.rawfoodinfo.com/articles/art_arewe treatingcancerbutkillingpatient.htm>.

[4]   *The Beautiful Truth*, dir. Steve Kroschel, Documentary, 2008.

[5]   "Gerson Institute Healing with Nature," <http://gerson.org/Programs/ findgersonclinic.htm>.

[6]   Helena Reimer, "The Gerson Institute," <http://www.ezinearticles.com /?The-Gerson-Institute&id=3494956>.

[7]   Michael Lerner, "Choices In Healing: Integrating the Best of Conventional and Complementary Approaches to Cancer," <http://www.commonweal.org/ pubs/ choices/4.html>.

[8]   *Healing Cancer from the Inside Out*, dir. Mike Anderson, DVD. 2008).

[9]   Lerner.

[10] Andrew Scholberg, "Reagan's cancer treated in Germany," <http:// freegrab. net/Reagan%27s%20cancer%20treated%20in%20Germany.htm >.

[11] *Healing Cancer from the Inside Out*, dir. Mike Anderson, DVD. 2008).

Friday, January 8, 2010

11. Don't Be "Led Down the Primrose Path"

The oncologist may hand you the drug information booklet (as is legally required), and then tell you not to read the information too closely because it may scare you. Do not be led down the primrose path. Read the booklet. Believe the description of side effects. Don't believe it when the doctor tries to minimize the side effects. The side effects are very real, and some are permanent. You will be administered "the maximum sub-lethal dosage that the body can handle." Who would possibly want to agree to take a sub-lethal dose of anything? Only someone who was led to that point by desperation and fear. What happens if a mistake is made with the dosage, or if your body can't handle a "maximum sub-lethal dose"? Will you receive a lethal injection? For what crime: You didn't do your homework? You trusted your doctor? Don't rush into treatment, you have time to review all your options. Insist upon it. It is *your* life. It is *your* choice.

In a survey of oncologists conducted at McGill University Cancer Center in Canada, 81% responded that they themselves would not take Cisplatin (a common chemotherapy treatment), and 75% responded that they would refuse any type of chemotherapy, citing the "ineffectiveness of chemotherapy and its unacceptable degree of toxicity."[1]

People must be offered the freedom of choice. The "standard of care" is a cookie-cutter, "one size fits all" approach. Educate yourself, be comfortable with your choice. For some cancers, chemo may be the correct choice, but don't let it be your knee-jerk reaction choice. Choose wisely.

Ask the questions, "what else do you offer?", "what other options are there?" If the response is "that's it, that *is* the only option," then get a second opinion, and a third and a fourth, until you are comfortable with the option of your choosing. Your choices in this challenge are literally a life and death decision. Don't be afraid to challenge a medical recommendation. Understand the circular reasoning of the orthodox "standard of care": there are *no* other options for a traditional oncologist to offer, because all other options have been suppressed by traditional oncology. Do not accept this situation; this is bad medicine.

Don't be "led down the primrose path." *That* is not the way to wellness. Choose the path to health through truth and inspiration. *This* is the way to wellness.

---

[1] Dr. George J Georgiou, Ph.D.,ND.,D.Sc (AM), "Are we treating cancer, but killing the patient?",<http://www.rawfoodinfo.com/articles/ art_arewe treatingcancerbutkillingpatient.htm>.

Friday, January 8, 2010

12. Intention

These vignettes are an expression of my personal experience. I am not a professional researcher or a medical professional. The intention is to be thought-provoking, to encourage people to research and educate themselves prior to accepting the "standard of care" treatment. I believe that every person is ultimately responsible for their own health care decisions. It is your decision whether or not you will "just say no to chemo."

My catalyst was the fact that I was almost sentenced to death by chemo. The cancer industry is "in too deep" to admit that they are wrong; they continue to perpetuate the myth, and they continue to harm and kill hundreds of thousands of Americans every year with ineffective, experimental, and expensive "treatments."

Chemotherapy can cause other cancers. This is something that people are not told unless they ask. I asked. The oncologist confirmed it. When I tell people this, they are shocked. I have since read, in *Beating Cancer with Nutrition* written by the former nutrition director at Cancer Treatment Centers of America, that the risk of chemo causing leukemia in ovarian cancer patients far outweighs any possible benefit.[1] Do ovarian cancer patients know that they are trading one form of cancer for another when they sign up for chemotherapy? Probably not.

When the oncologist recommends "precautionary chemo," and says that, with chemo you have a 30% chance of recurrence, and if it does recur, you probably will not survive five (5) years, and if you don't have chemo, then the chance of recurrence is higher, then that is the time to start asking questions.

"How much higher?" I asked.

"Higher."

"Yes, but how much higher?"

"Higher."

I could not understand why I wasn't getting a straight answer. That statistic should have been at the tip of the tongue. The reason it wasn't at the tip of the tongue is because that statistic simply does not exist. It is not known if that number is actually higher, *or* maybe it is actually lower! When you are in that position, you are *very* vulnerable, as I was. I had my "meltdown" when I went for a consultation at a center that markets itself as "a place for hope." I walked in feeling hopeful and walked out feeling hopeless. In the evening after I was handed my death sentence there, I very fortuitously met an ancillary staff person who told me how the cancer statistics are compiled by SEER: that the "current" statistics are almost five (5) years old and that there is no control group, making the statistics essentially meaningless to any individual. He told me not to believe the statistics. When I received a similar dire prognosis and the same medical recommendation for "precautionary chemotherapy" in another oncologist's office, the nurse told me that I didn't need chemo. I was puzzled that I was being told to disregard the doctors' recommendation by these honest people, but this felt like truth, and it empowered me.

Ask questions. Ask to see the statistics. I did, and was brushed off. Insist upon it. Ask to see studies. I did, and was told that there were no studies to support the recommended treatment for me. Demand answers.

My intention is to raise enough reasonable doubt about the effectiveness of chemotherapy to get people to pause, research, educate themselves, participate in their own health care, explore other options on their own, and then make an *informed* decision, based upon truthful, factual information, and not on the skewed statistics presented by the pharmaceutical companies. The first two (2) oncologists I saw were parroting drug salesmen's pitches. The third oncologist was truthful, and said that it is not known whether or not it matters if people start chemo right after surgery, or if they wait six (6) months. It is just not known.

There is no urgency. People do not have to rush into it. People have time to think and educate themselves.

People have a right to know the truth, and they also have a right to choose non-toxic solutions. Non-toxic solutions have been systematically suppressed by the FDA, and people need to start demanding alternatives.

It has been ingrained in all of us that a pill can solve all our problems. That is western medicine; that is the American way. Check it out, you have the time. But most people do not check it out, especially if it is not a personal issue with them. Even if it is a personal issue, most people do not check it out. They have been brainwashed to believe in the myth of chemotherapy.

Every day, I thank God and my husband that I checked it out. It is my intention to live. This is truth. Insist that it be told. Ask questions and demand truthful answers. Your life depends on it. This is the only way to wellness.

---

[1]   Patrick Quillen, PhD, *Beating Cancer with Nutrition* (Carlsbad, CA: Nutrition Times Press, Inc., 2005).

Saturday, January 9, 2010

13. Chemo-Gate

A systematic suppression of legitimate proven or potential cancer cures by the cancer industry and all of the participants of that industry has been carried out for years, all in the name of protecting the public.

Twenty-five years ago, in January 1986, the suppression was brought to light in testimony presented to the United States Congress. Mary Yevchak testified that she was forced to undergo chemotherapy treatment which almost killed her, and she had to leave this country to seek the non-toxic treatment which cured her. She traveled to the Immuno-Augmentative Therapy Clinic in Freeport, Bahamas in April 1984, and spent two (2) months receiving the treatment that eliminated the cancer from her body.[1] Still, over twenty-five years later, our country is still pushing toxic treatments that do *not* work, and suppressing non-toxic treatments that *do* work. We need to bring the term "chemo-gate" into the vernacular. Chemo-gate must be exposed. Where are the Bob Woodwards and Carl Bernsteins of this age? The mainstream media will not pick up this story because of the potential loss of massive advertising revenues from Big Pharma. People don't talk about it, or if they do, they talk about it in hushed tones. It is up to the thousands of people who are aware of this travesty to start talking about it. Now. Openly.

There have been Orwellian "revolutionaries" who tell the truth. According to Dr. Linus Pauling, Nobel Laureate, "Everyone should know that the 'war on cancer' is largely a fraud."[2] In 1975, Dr. James Watson (Nobel Prize winner for determining the shape of DNA, and former Board member of the National Cancer Advisory Board) was asked about the National Cancer Program, and he proclaimed, "It's a bunch of shit," and that "the American public is being sold a nasty bill of goods."[3] More recently, in 2009, Dr. Watson was quoted as saying that the National Cancer Institute (NCI) is "a largely rudderless ship in dire need of a bold captain."[4] Barry Lynes, in his book *The Healing of Cancer, The Cures-The Cover-ups and the Solution Now!*, discusses the 1953 Senate Investigation chaired by Senator Charles Tobey, which reported that a conspiracy existed to suppress effective cancer treatments. Fortunately for the accused conspirators, Senator Tobey died of an "apparent" heart attack, and the investigation ended with his death. Lynes also reported on the court case involving the falsification of records by the Food and Drug Administration (FDA), which as early as 1964 was intent upon stopping alternative cancer treatments which had cured cancer patients. Lynes also uncovered the practice of two (2) New York City doctors, one of whom was associated with Sloan-Kettering, who intentionally injected unknowing patients with live cancer cells in an experiment. The doctors were placed on probation for a year, while the whistle-blowers were fired. Lynes further reports that in 1977, an investigative team from Newsday, a Long Island, New York daily newspaper, found "serious conflicts of interest" at the National Cancer Institute (NCI). Also, Lynes notes that the Congressional hearings held in 1986 revealed an NCI-organized cover-up of an effective alternative cancer treatment.

According to Lynes, "The cancer establishment now has a 50-year history of vast corruption, incompetence, and organized suppression of cancer therapies which actually work. Millions of people have suffered terrible torture and death because those in charge took payoffs, played it safe, had closed minds to the innovative, or simply were afraid to do what was obviously and morally right . . ."[5]

In 1981, the National Cancer Institute abolished the NCI research on the development of antitumor agents from plants. Not only did the direction move away from researching the beneficial effects of non-toxic treatments that have demonstrated effectiveness against specific cancers, but the FDA has taken this approach even further, by actually banning "entire species, even genus, of cancer-fighting herbs. We don't just mean individual products. In some cases, we mean the entire genus of plant, scrub, even tree. In some cases, the 'outlaw plant,' had a centuries-old, proven history of effectiveness. Mysteriously, any plant that has shown strong anti-cancer properties has been removed from store shelves and placed on 'blacklists.' And yet the plants that have been banned are those which exhibit the most promise and are empirically the most effective when properly processed. These plants are not banned by legislatures. There are no laws enforcing such bans. These are 'policy directives,' bureaucratic decisions made without any input from the electorate or members of the everyday practicing health care community. These decisions are made by government workers with close ties to the pharmaceutical industry. There is no accountability to the electorate, only to large corporations whose profits in such obscene practices as radiation and chemotherapy treatment must be protected as all costs."[6]

In 2009, the FDA posted on their website a list of "187 Fake Cancer "Cures" Consumers Should Avoid."[7] Ironically, the director of the FDA's Office of Enforcement said that these products are dangerous "because they could prevent a patient from seeking proper treatment for cancer. They could also harm a cancer patient by interacting with other drugs the patient is taking. Health fraud is a 'cruel form of greed,' [calling] fraud involving cancer treatment 'especially heartless.'"[8] The irony of the FDA's statement should not be lost on all those taken in by the cruel, heartless, greedy fraud of chemotherapy. Paradoxically, the FDA proclaims chemotherapy toxic drug treatments as "safe and effective," despite the fact that a common side effect is death. The cause of death is commonly attributed by the medical profession to *cancer*, and not to *chemotherapy*. *If* the cause of death is attributed to chemotherapy, it is termed as "an overreaction" to chemotherapy.[9] This is the "blame the patient" syndrome: a clever and effective move to sidestep liability.

Chemo-gate must be exposed. "There is a cancer growing on the Presidency" (John Dean, 1973). There is a cancer growing on the cancer industry. This is truth.

---

[1] James, David. "A Last Stand, An American Tragedy. Testimony of Mary and Michael Yevchak, Congressional Public Hearing," <http://www.cancercontrolinfo.com/ index2B.html>.

[2] <http://www.healingcancernaturally.com>.

[3] *Healing Cancer from the Inside Out*, dir. Mike Anderson, DVD, 2008).

[4] "National Cancer Institute a 'rudderless ship',"<http://www.psa-rising.com/blog/2009/08/national-cancer-institute-a-rudderless-ship/>.

[5] Barry Lynes, From the Introduction to *The Healing of Cancer, The Cures-The Cover-ups and the Solution Now!*, <http://health.centreforce.com/ health/industry.html>.

[6] "Cancerolytic Herbs: a History of Suppression," <http://health.centreforce.com/health/industry.html>.

[7] "FDA: 187 Fake Cancer "Cures" Consumers Should Avoid." <http://www.fda.gov/Drugs/GuidanceComplianceRegulatoryInformation/Enforcement ActivitiesbyFDA/ucm171057.htm>.

[8] "FDA Warns of Internet Sales of Fake Cancer Cures," <http://www.healthnews.com/alerts-outbreaks/fda-warns-against-internet-sales-fake-cancer-cures-1257.html>.

[9] *Healing Cancer from the Inside Out*, dir. Mike Anderson, DVD, 2008).

Sunday, January 10, 2010

14. Chemo: The Cash Cow of the Cancer Industry

"In business, a cash cow is a product or a business unit that generates unusually high profit margins: so high that it is responsible for a large amount of a company's operating profit. This profit far exceeds the amount necessary to maintain the cash cow business."[1]

A firm is characterized as a "cash cow" when the firm is not investing in product improvements. This could be the case if a company believes that the future of a product line is threatened as a result of another product potentially eroding its market share. An operational risk of a "cash cow" business is complacency, with management ignoring the need to adapt to changing market conditions.

Every business searches for a cash cow product: a product that yields a high profit margin and requires low investment costs. The term "cash cow" originated as a comparison to a dairy cow that can be continually milked with very low maintenance.

Chemo is the "cash cow of the cancer industry." However, as the cancer industry controls and monopolizes the market through the cooperation of complicit regulatory and research agencies, there *are* no market forces present; the industry operates essentially as a monopoly, in a vacuum, and any potential challenges are suppressed by the regulatory agencies. Competing natural, non-toxic products are either banned from entering the marketplace, or are denigrated by the FDA. Obscene profits continue to roll in on the backs of deceived cancer patients. The cancer industry is insulated from the normal forces of the marketplace, which, if allowed to exist, would force it to: 1) recall all chemotherapy products as unsafe; and 2) introduce safer products into the marketplace. It is time to put the chemo cash cow out to pasture. The milk is sour.

Demand accountability. Demand the truth. Demand access to treatments that are beneficial. Demand that insurance companies start covering beneficial treatments, and stop wasting money on ineffective chemotherapy that has not been proven to cure cancer. Insurance coverage validates chemo, because people believe that if insurance covers the treatment, then the treatment must work. But the insurance money only serves to feed the cash cow, it keeps the cancer industry fat; it has little to do with how well the treatment works.

Demand our rights to make our own choices in our own health care. Demand the truth. This is the only way to wellness.

---

[1]   Wikipedia, ‹http://en.wikipedia.org›.

Tuesday, January 12, 2010

15. It's Illegal to Buy Vitamin B-17 in America

Vitamin B-17, or Laetrile, is banned in the U.S. Laetrile is a modified form of amygdalin, a naturally-occurring substance found in apricots, peaches, and almonds. It is just incredible that U.S. citizens cannot buy a vitamin in this country.

An article called *Jason Vale and the Cancer Mafia* tells the story of someone who was prosecuted and jailed for selling apricot seeds. Jason Vale cured his cancer with apricot seeds, and felt he should help others cure themselves as well. Vale was selling apricot seeds and promoting them as a cancer cure. The FDA issued a cease and desist order, which Vale ignored and as a result, was jailed. Despite the fact that this natural treatment is effective, the FDA not surprisingly sided with the pharmaceutical companies in determining that this vitamin should be banned. The pharmaceutical companies cannot patent natural substances, and therefore, cannot make money on Vitamin B-17. Consequently, any challenge to the profit-making chemotherapy drugs must be eliminated. The article states that it is the mission of government agencies and foundations to "research cures and treatments for cancer, not to focus on protecting their significant financial interest." However, according to this article, the priority has been, and will continue to be, on the bottom line: "Laetrile and all other natural products, used in treating cancer are a threat to their [the cancer industry's] profits." [1]

Pressure must be exerted upon the FDA to allow U.S. citizens to exercise our civil liberties in choosing our own health care. Non-toxic treatments are banned; toxic treatments are routinely prescribed. The truth must be revealed to enable people to discover the way to wellness. We must demand it.

---

[1]   "Jason Vale and the Cancer Mafia," <<http://www.apricotsfromgod.info/ jvale/>>.

Saturday, January 16, 2010

16. The Dorothy Revelations

Dorothy Brennan was my father's second wife. She died in 1995 after extensive chemotherapy sessions. She was diagnosed with breast cancer, had the radical mastectomy recommended back in those radical days, had the recommended chemotherapy: the "standard of care." The cancer survived and moved to the liver. Dorothy continued the recommended treatments and she did not survive it.

Janet Taylor Rizzolo was my wonderful friend for thirty years. Years ago, she was tagged with the nickname "Dorothy." She died in 2006 after extensive chemotherapy sessions. She had been diagnosed with breast cancer, had the recommended surgeries, had the recommended chemotherapy: the "standard of care." The cancer survived and moved to the liver. She underwent "experimental" chemotherapy. Taylor ("Dorothy") continued the recommended treatments and she did not survive it.

When I first started my very strange odyssey, I asked God and my spiritual guides for advice about taking chemotherapy, and one night in a dream, I heard Taylor's voice say, very simply, "Don't do it, Margaret." It was very powerful, and I awoke from a sound sleep. Last night during a Reiki session, again I heard Taylor say again, very simply, "Don't do it, Margaret." And then Dorothy Brennan joined in, and collectively, they said, "It killed us. We thought that we were doing the right thing." And with that, I had the realization that together they gave me the answer I needed and guided me onto the right path, and are working through me to let others know that they must question conventional treatment.

I love these two women. They both loved life; both were very intelligent, well-read, strong, funny, giving, generous, engaged and engaging women. Both were very concerned about the well-being of others. And they are both still very concerned about the well-being of others, and continue to do their work from where they are. I am simply the conduit to help reveal the truth. They have been my inspiration on my way to wellness.

Saturday, January 16, 2010

17. Cancer Is Not a Death Sentence—Chemo Is

A meta-analysis conducted by three (3) oncologists published in *Clinical Oncology* entitled "The Contribution of Cytotoxic Chemotherapy to 5-year Survival in Adult Malignancies" examined the benefit of chemotherapy in the treatment of adults with common cancers. The study examined the results of all clinical trials conducted in Australia and the United States from 1990 to 2004 that reported a "statistically significant increase in 5-year survival due to the use of chemotherapy in adult malignancies." The results of the meta-analysis revealed that chemotherapy is effective in contributing to just over 2% improved 5-year survival rates in cancer patients.[1] This is the blended rate for all the common cancers examined in the study. Chemo has a 0% effectiveness rate for site-specific cancers such as bladder, kidney, pancreas, prostate, and uterus, and for other cancers such as melanoma and sarcoma. Chemo has an effectiveness rate of 1.4% for breast cancer; 3.7% for brain cancer; 8.9% for ovarian cancer. The effectiveness rate is 37.7% for testicular cancer and 40.3% Hodgkins Disease;[2] these outliers drive *up* the effectiveness rate of chemo to just over 2%.

The website, "Because YOU need the right info to make the right decision . . ." states that, "Chemo has almost a 98% fatality rate."[3] *That* sentence is the most important sentence you will ever read. This article also discusses the *Clinical Oncology* study, which, notably, was conducted in Australia; any study that reveals the truth is suppressed in the U.S. by the FDA and Big Pharma. The results of the study indicate that only 2.1% of Americans receiving chemotherapy will survive for 5 (five) years after they have been diagnosed.[4] The converse, of course, is that 97.9% of all people in the U.S. who receive chemotherapy will *die within five years* after diagnosis and toxic treatment! People feel that when they are ill, they must take some kind of medicine. Sometimes the best action is no action. There *are* healthy, beneficial alternatives. Find them. Cancer is not a death sentence. Chemotherapy is.

The Chemofraud.com website states that the "CONCEPT OF 'CHEMOTHERAPY SUCCESS' IS LARGELY A FRAUD . . . the fact is that cancer patients often die from the drugs themselves due to toxicity. Cancer patients deserve to know the truth and to make choices based upon this truth. And the truth is that the proven cancer prevention strategies and the real cures for cancer do not need a prescription, nor do they require surgery or barbaric procedures like radiation or chemotherapy."[5]

The website quotes several cancer specialists. Dr. Glenn Warner, one of the most highly qualified cancer specialists in the United States, used alternative treatments on his cancer patients with great success. On the treatment of cancer in this country he said: *"We have a multi-billion dollar industry that is killing people, right and left, just for financial gain. Their idea of research is to see whether two doses of this poison is better than three doses of that poison."*

Dr. Alan C. Nixon, past president of the American Chemical Society writes, *"As a chemist trained to interpret data, it is incomprehensible to me that physicians can ignore the clear evidence that chemotherapy does much, much more harm than good."* Dr. Charles Mathe, French cancer specialist, states, *"If I contracted cancer, I would never go to a standard cancer treatment centre. Only cancer victims who live far from such centres have a chance. Yet, day after day, year after year, the Cancer Industry continues to put these toxic chemicals into the bodies of cancer patients. And the patients let them do it, even volunteering for new 'guinea pig' studies, simply because someone with a degree from a school of disease (also known as medical school) told them it was their 'only option.' It costs lots of money for them to poison the body of cancer patients, and the patients gladly pay it. Sadly, some people will spend six figures a year poisoning their bodies because their 'doctor told them to do it.' The truth is that there are many effective natural cancer treatments that don't require a barbaric procedure like chemotherapy."* [6]

I was an early supporter of chemotherapy. My own mother was diagnosed with breast cancer in 1992, and participated in the tamoxifen trials. At the time, I was proud of my mother for being a pioneer. I realize now that she was a pawn of Big Pharma, and I am amazed that she survived chemotherapy treatment. I don't recall at the time that she was advised that tamoxifen could cause uterine cancer, which is now listed as a possible side effect.[7]

My mother survived her cancer, but almost twenty (20) years later is affected by idiopathic Parkinson's Disease (PD), a "degenerative disorder of the central nervous system that often impairs the sufferer's motor skills, speech, and other functions."[8] Idiopathic Parkinson's Disease is a "type of parkinsonism for which there is no known cause ("idiopathic" = of unknown origin). This is the most common type of parkinsonism (unlike parkinsonism caused by a known toxin, repeated trauma, or certain drugs)."[9]

My guess is that my mother's PD is not idiopathic at all; that it is a direct result of chemotherapy and her five (5) year participation in the tamoxifen trials, during which she experienced neuropathy. You cannot continually stress the central nervous system without inflicting long-term damage. It is my opinion that my mother's "idiopathic Parkinson's Disease" was the long-term collateral damage inflicted by chemotherapy. People should know the truth.

Pay attention to the sign posts along the way to wellness. Experts are speaking out against chemotherapy. These are educated, knowledgeable, and brave people. Listen to them. Chemotherapy does not work. It is *not* the way to wellness. It is *not* truth.

---

[1] Dr. George J Georgiou, Ph.D.,ND.,D.Sc (AM), "Are we treating cancer, but killing the patient?",<http://www.rawfoodinfo.com/articles/art_ arewetreating cancerbutkillingpatient.htm>.

[2] *Healing Cancer from the Inside Out*, dir. Mike Anderson, DVD, 2008).

[3,4,5,6] "Because you need the right info to make the right decision," <http://www. ChemoFraud.com>.

[7] "National Cancer Institute Factsheet," <http://www.cancer.gov/cancer topics/ factsheet/Therapy/tamoxifen>.

[8] Wikipedia, <http://en.Wikipedia.org>.

[9] "Redwood Caregiver Resource Center," <http://www.redwoodcrc.org /fact Sheets/Parkinsons/XGlossaryOfTerms.doc>.

Saturday, January 30, 2010

18. Tribute to Taylor

Today is my dear friend Taylor's birthday. She would have been 59 today. I dedicate this day to her: To Taylor, on your birthday, with love and gratitude.

Taylor battled chemotherapy and told me toward the end of her battle that she had "two days in the past year and a half when I felt OK, not great, not even good, but just OK. The rest of the time I felt like shit." This is a real person, a human being, not just a statistic. She died by following medical advice. Would she still be alive if she hadn't? We need to recognize that there are millions of human beings, real people, like Taylor, who should have had better options presented to them and who could have had better outcomes.

The most important quality a person could have, according to Taylor, was kindness. Within each act of kindness was a lesson, teaching others how to be kind. She loved to laugh; she had a great wit; she loved life. I think of Taylor often, and I am inspired to do what she would do: talk to a stranger, call a friend, make someone smile or laugh, and take every opportunity to be kind to someone. She was a wonderful friend and an amazing human being. But most of all, her life was kind. Her death was not.

Happy Birthday Taylor. I wish I knew then what I know now. Truth. It may have helped you find your way to wellness. You are *my* inspiration to find my way to wellness.

My birthday song to you:

> *"May your strength give us strength,*
> *May your faith give us faith,*
> *May your hope give us hope,*
> *May your love give us love."*
> ~Bruce Springsteen

Sunday, January 31, 2010

19. Chemo-"therapy": The Oxymoron

Chemo + Therapy? Hardly. Toxic chemicals are not therapy for disease. Chemo as "therapy" is a fallacy, a myth, an unintended oxymoron, a "contradiction in terms."

Madison Cavanaugh refers to the Pharmaceutical industry as a "cartel."[1] A cartel is "a group of businesses that collude to limit competition within an industry or market."[2] Very simple natural cures that have been used for over 160 years in the Far East have been suppressed by the pharmaceutical-medical complex, a complex as insidious as the military-industrial complex suspected in the JFK assassination. This is a chemical conspiracy driven hard by the pharmaceutical cartel. Just try watching your TV at night without viewing a single drug ad—impossible! This cartel is in your living room every night, convincing you that you are ill, and that you need to buy their products. Do what I do: hit the mute button or leave the room. We, the people, do not need to buy these drugs. We, the people, need to unite to fight for our health freedom. When I was growing up, I was taught that censorship and suppression was prevalent in Communist Russia, but America was the "Land of the Free." Apparently, not so. As we, Baby Boomers, age out and experience various health issues, we are the new targets of Big Pharma. Big Pharma already has our parents on fistfuls of prescription drugs, causing side effects for which (of course) even more drugs are prescribed. Our parents' generation apparently does not practice what they preached: "Just say no to drugs." We Baby Boomers are more and more susceptible to health information, misinformation, disinformation, and health care suppression. We need to protest this suppression, just as we protested the Vietnam War, Watergate, and the treatment of migrant workers.

Seven (7) states have "Health Freedom Laws": New Mexico, Arizona, Louisiana, Rhode Island, California, Minnesota, Oklahoma. Why do we need laws to guarantee and protect our right to Health Freedom? The National Health Freedom Coalition's mission as stated is:

> "To promote access to all health care information, services, treatments and products that the people deem beneficial for their own health, healing, well-being and survival; and to promote the health of the people of this nation. Consumers are in jeopardy of losing access to holistic health care practitioners. Medical doctors, dentists, homeopaths, naturopaths, and alternative practitioners across the country are being harassed, investigated, and detained for their actions!" Why? Because practitioners are presenting a health care

option to consumers that is different from conventional medicine and are practicing a holistic approach that involves natural substances and techniques. Because of restrictive state practitioner laws, these individuals can lose their licenses or be prosecuted for practicing medicine without a license. Access to dietary supplements, health care products and devices is at risk. Manufacturers are investigated by federal agencies such as FDA and FTC or local authorities for making health claims for products that are therapeutic in nature, even when the claims are truthful and not misleading. This censorship must stop. Global guidelines and trade agreements are being passed that will impact our access to many products that we appreciate and depend on for maintaining our health. National Health Freedom Coalition works to protect the right of all people to access their favorite health care practitioners and health care products, as well as to protect the right to access many other healing arts services that really resonate with people's path to wellness!" [3]

As a nation, we must demand Health Freedom: freedom to access truthful information, and freedom to choose non-toxic health options. Chemo is *not* therapy. It is not the truth. It is not the way to wellness.

---

[1]   Madison Cavanaugh, *The One-Minute Cure: The Secret to Healing Virtually all Diseases* (Beverly Hills: Think-Outside-the-Book Publishing, Inc., 2008).

[2]   <http://www.wiktionary.org>.

[3]   "National Health Freedom Action," <http://www.nationalhealthfreedom. org/>.

Saturday, February 6, 2010

20. Rise Up . . .

The Pray for the Cure e-mail continued to circulate, and in response, I was inspired to write my own "prayer."

—Original Message—

To: mbermel
From: ed
Date: Saturday, February 6, 2010, 4:00 p.m.
Subject: Fw: Please do this

93% won't forward
A small request . . . Just one line
Dear God, I pray for a cure for cancer. Amen
All you are asked to do is keep this circulating, even if it's only to one more person.
In memory of anyone you know who has been struck down by cancer or is still living with it.

—Original Message—
From: mbermel
Date: Saturday, February 6, 2010, 5:39 p.m.
Subject: Rise Up . . .
To: ed

Please send this in response to the "Pray for the Cure" email, which only serves to perpetuate the myth that "the cure is right around the corner." The cures are already here. Rise up and demand them.

My prayer is in memory of anyone you know who has suffered through chemotherapy.

Dear God,

I pray that the natural cures for cancer will no longer be suppressed by the FDA.

I pray that the medical "standard of care" will be expanded beyond surgery, radiation, and chemotherapy to include natural, non-toxic treatments that actually benefit the patient.

I pray that the toxic solutions which are embraced by the cancer industry be acknowledged as the medical failures that they are.

I pray that the pharmaceutical industry, whose only interest is their bottom line, will stop monopolizing the cancer market with toxic, poisonous "treatments" which often do more harm than good.

I pray that people will come to learn the true motive of the pharmaceutical companies: the profit motive.

I pray that people will learn that because natural cures cannot be patented, they cannot make money for the cancer industry, and thus they are suppressed, dismissed, and ridiculed even though they are beneficial.

I pray that oncologists stop scaring patients into chemotherapy treatment: sometimes the medicine is worse than the disease.

I pray that people start to understand that their loved ones are dying from chemotherapy, and not from "cancer."

I pray that this message reaches the consciousness of the general public, so that people do not continue to march with resignation into the chemotherapy infusion chambers just to die a slow, painful death.

I pray that people will believe that treatment for this disease does not have to be fatal.

I pray that the public starts to question and research the "standard of care," and then demand that the cures for cancer which have already been proven to work, will become openly available to those people who choose them.

I pray that people will demand their right to know, and then demand their right to choose.

Amen.

Just say no to chemo. This is truth and inspiration, and the way to wellness.

Wednesday, February 17, 2010

21. Big Brother

A February 17th cannot pass by without pausing to remember my brother Jack. I think of him every day of my life, but this date holds very special significance: this was the day that my father was born in 1925 and it was the day that my brother died suddenly in 2002. Jack's death was a medical statistic, his was one of 195,000 annual preventable "in-hospital deaths from medical errors" in the United States (HealthGrades, 2004).[1] He was a good patient, believed the doctors, and followed medical recommendations. Jack was a runner, a world-class marathoner, and ran in the 1980 Olympic time trials. He was in excellent condition. For that reason, the doctors dismissed his physical complaints.

Jack's death was the most significant event in my life. His death almost killed me. I internalized his loss, and the ever-present grief manifested in my disease.

My first awareness of life included Jack's presence. I had never known life without Jack. During grade school, Jack was the altar boy for the daily 7:30 a.m. masses at the Chapel School convent. He was the first one out of the house. On snowy mornings, his footprints would lead a path from our front steps to the steps of the convent. As the oldest of six (6) children, Jack had the best pair of boots in the house. I would wear my mother's shoe boots which were a few sizes too big for me, but they worked in the deep snow, as long as I stayed in Jack's footprints. Once I passed the convent, I was on my own. But I always set out, reassured that I was following Jack, hoping, if I walked fast enough, to catch up to him. These snowy morning treks became a metaphor for my life—following in Jack's footprints, never being able to catch up to him, but confident that I was on the right path. As I went through grade school, I realized at the beginning of every school year that great things were expected of me because Jack was my brother. The bar had been set very high.

Jack expected only one thing of his friends and family, and that was that they be the absolute best person that they were capable of being. He was instrumental in shaping my life; I discussed all of my major life decisions with him, and he always listened very patiently and gave me the absolute best advice.

He taught us the lessons he came to teach us. He expects my personal best effort in this situation. I know that his advice to me now would be to find out as much as I can about this situation, critically assess medical advice, and listen to my heart. His footprints are fading now. I will follow him someday, but not now. I still have life experiences that remain ahead for me, lessons to learn and lessons to teach. My work is not done here. But he is still leading me, and I am confident that I am on the right path. After his death, I very often found a feather on my path, and often in an unexpected place. To me, the feather became the sign of Jack's presence, the sign that I was on the right path.

I am on the way to wellness, by discovering truth and inspiration. And on this labyrinthine path, this cancer odyssey, I am becoming the absolute best person I am capable of being. My big brother expects nothing less. Truth. Inspiration.

---

[1] "In-Hospital Deaths from Medical Errors at 195,000 per year, HealthGrades Study Finds," <http://www.healthgrades.com/media/DMS/pdf/ InhosptialDeaths PatientSafetyPressRelease072704.pdf. [sic]

Friday, February 26, 2010

22. The Establishment Comes Clean (or Not)

There is an e-mail circulating which cites an established medical institution as the source of an article which *finally* reveals the truth about cancer: that the conventional treatments do not work. However, that institution credited with the e-mail has disclaimed the article and proclaimed it to be a hoax. So the hope that the establishment was coming clean has been extinguished; the establishment is *not* coming clean, the hoax of chemotherapy is still perpetuated by mainstream oncology. Someday the cancer business arm of the medical oncology profession will focus on healing people instead of leading them to certain death. That is my hope. Although the author of this e-mail is unknown, the truth of the article is recognized. I believe that the intent of the author was to validate the truth. But "truth is truth" (Shakespeare) and can stand alone.

" . . . CHEMO . . . CANCER

AFTER YEARS OF TELLING PEOPLE CHEMOTHERAPY IS THE ONLY WAY TO TRY ("TRY, BEING THE KEY WORD) TO ELIMINATE CANCER, [a medical institution] IS FINALLY STARTING TO TELL YOU THERE IS AN ALTERNATIVE WAY.

Cancer Update

1. Every person has cancer cells in the body. These cancer cells do not show up in the standard tests until they have multiplied to a few billion. When doctors tell cancer patients that there are no more cancer cells in their bodies after treatment, it just means the tests are unable to detect the cancer cells because they have not reached the detectable size.
2. [A critical mass of] cancer cells occur between 6 to more than 10 times in a person's lifetime.
3. When the person's immune system is strong, the cancer cells will be destroyed and prevented from multiplying and forming tumors.
4. When a person has cancer, it indicates the person has multiple nutritional deficiencies. These could be due to genetic, environmental, food and lifestyle factors.
5. To overcome the multiple nutritional deficiencies, changing diet and including supplements will strengthen the immune system.

6. Chemotherapy involves poisoning the rapidly-growing cancer cells and also destroys rapidly-growing healthy cells in the bone marrow, gastrointestinal tract etc, and can cause organ damage, to liver, kidneys, heart, lungs, etc.
7. Radiation, while destroying cancer cells, also burns, scars and damages healthy cells, tissues and organs.
8. Initial treatment with chemotherapy and radiation will often reduce tumor size. However, prolonged use of chemotherapy and radiation do not result in more tumor destruction.
9. When the body has too much toxic burden from chemotherapy and radiation, the immune system is either compromised or destroyed; hence, the person can succumb to various kinds of infections and complications.
10. Chemotherapy and radiation can cause cancer cells to mutate and become resistant and difficult to destroy. Surgery can also cause cancer cells to spread to other sites.
11. An effective way to battle cancer is to starve the cancer cells by not feeding it with the foods it needs to multiply.

CANCER CELLS FEED ON:

a. Sugar is a cancer-feeder. By cutting off sugar it cuts off one important food supply to the cancer cells. Sugar substitutes like NutraSweet, Equal, Spoonful, etc., are made with Aspartame which is harmful. A better natural substitute would be Manuka honey or molasses but only in very small amounts. Table salt has a chemical added to make it white in color. Better alternative is Bragg's aminos or sea salt.
b. Milk causes the body to produce mucus, especially in the gastrointestinal tract. Cancer feeds on mucus. By cutting off milk and substituting with unsweetened soy milk, cancer cells are being starved.
c. Cancer cells thrive in an acid environment. A meat-based diet is acidic and it is best to eat fish, and a little chicken rather than beef or pork. Meat also contains livestock antibiotics, growth hormones and parasites, which are all harmful, especially to people with cancer.
d. A diet made of 80% fresh vegetables and juice, whole grains, seeds, nuts and a little fruit help put the body into an alkaline environment. Fresh vegetable juices provide live enzymes that are easily absorbed and reach down to cellular levels within 15 minutes of consumption to nourish and enhance growth of healthy cells. To obtain live enzymes for building healthy cells try and drink fresh vegetable juice (most vegetables including bean sprouts) and eat some raw vegetables 2 or

3 times a day. Enzymes are destroyed at temperatures of 104 degrees F (40 degrees C).

e. Avoid coffee, tea, and chocolate, which have high caffeine. Green tea is a better alternative and has cancer fighting properties. Drink purified or filtered water, to avoid known toxins and heavy metals in tap water. Distilled water is acidic, avoid it.

f. Meat protein is difficult to digest and requires a lot of digestive enzymes. Undigested meat remaining in the intestines become putrified and leads to more toxic buildup.

g. Cancer cell walls have a tough protein covering. By refraining from or eating less meat it frees more enzymes to attack the protein walls of cancer cells and allows the body's killer cells to destroy the cancer cells.

h. Some supplements build up the immune system (IP6, Flor-essence, Essiac, antioxidants, vitamins, minerals, EFAs, etc.) enabling the body's own killer cells to destroy cancer cells. Other supplements like Vitamin E are known to cause apoptosis, or programmed cell death, which is the body's normal method of disposing of damaged, unwanted, or unneeded cells.

i. Cancer is a disease of the mind, body, and spirit. A proactive and positive spirit will help the cancer warrior be a survivor. Anger, unforgiveness and bitterness put the body into a stressful and acidic environment. Learn to have a loving and forgiving spirit. Learn to relax and enjoy life.

j. Cancer cells cannot thrive in an oxygenated environment. Exercising daily and deep breathing helps to get more oxygen down to the cellular level. Oxygen therapy is another means used to destroy cancer cells."

The e-mail continues on with a warning about the use of plastics in food storage and preparation. The website of the institution which is credited as the source of the e-mail has a point-by-point refutation. The website states that "traditional therapies, such as surgery, chemotherapy, and radiation therapy, work. The evidence is the millions of cancer survivors in the United States today who are alive because of these therapies. We recognize that treatments don't work in every patient, or sometimes work for a while and then stop working, and there are some cancers that are more difficult to cure than others." It also contends that "as part of a balanced diet, sugar, salt, milk, coffee, tea, meat, and chocolate—the foods the "Update" calls into question—are all safe choices . . ." The website also minimizes the effect of stress and state of mind on cancer recovery, essentially severing the mind-body connection. The website also states that "people are treated and completely cured of cancer everyday."[1] This is a surprising statement, as the conventional treatments endorsed by the website are never presented to a cancer patient as a "cure," and patients are not counted in the statistics as being "cured" until they have survived five (5) years from diagnosis. With statements such as these, the credibility of this website is questionable, and I have lost respect for the integrity of this medical institution.

There is truth in the Cancer Update e-mail, regardless of the denial by a major medical institution.

---

[1] "Cancer Update E-mail—It's a Hoax!," <*http://www. hopkinsmedicine.org/* kimmel_cancer_center/news_events/featured/cancer_ update_email_it_is_a_ hoax.html>.

Saturday, February 27, 2010

23. Natural Is Better

The pushing of drugs (chemo) for the treatment of symptoms of cancer is just the tip of the iceberg with Big Pharma. This mindset applies to every "disease" that exists.

Technically, "chemotherapy" is *any* chemical pharmaceutical, but the term has come into parlance as pertaining to the chemicals used to "treat" the symptoms of cancer. "Just say no to chemo."

An e-mail to my sister:

—Original Message—

From: mbermel
Date: Friday, February 26, 2010, 8:15 p.m.
Subject: Brain Health and Patient Rights
To: Patty

I had an appt today at a Preventive Medicine office that was highly recommended by a friend, a nutritionist, and an MD. The Nurse Practitioner said that at a conference she attended at Johns Hopkins, it was presented that ALL the drugs on the market now for Alzheimer's are ineffective. The belief is that Resveratrol IS effective, as it crosses the brain-blood barrier. Glaxo Smith Klein (GSK) bought out a smaller company for $720M last year that was researching Resveratrol, and GSK is working to synthesize a chemical resveratrol (because the naturally-occurring resveratrol cannot be patented, and thus the Pharma company cannot make money, so they have to re-create chemically a substance that already exists in nature). The following is an article from a website, which explains this in a little more detail.

"The research on the substance "Resveratrol" is exciting indeed. Now it has gotten the attention of the show 60 Minutes. It has been shown to optimize the aging process, extend healthy life, and be preventative for a variety of serious chronic degenerative diseases such as diabetes, heart disease, cancer, and Alzheimer's. Further, it is shown to enhance exercise performance, support healthy metabolism and support weight balancing. The research has all been done on the naturally occurring substance found in abundance in the skin of the red wine grape.

A substance that occurs in nature cannot be patented, so the drug company Glaxo Smith Kline is working on a synthetic version of Resveratrol, because the real thing is so exciting and the exclusive rights to the real thing cannot be owned and controlled. Researchers expect that a drug company will develop and sell a drug that contains the synthetic version of Resveratrol and make it available to the public, within our life time. What is even better is that the real thing is available now as a naturally occurring substance and in the form of a nutritional supplement, so the cost is low and no prescription is necessary."[1]

Big Pharma is on a mission, aided and abetted by the FDA, to turn naturally-occurring substances into chemically-compounded pharmaceuticals, to make money and eliminate the competition (vitamin/supplement companies). It is important to be aware that the motive is very simply, the *profit* motive.

This is not the first time that orthodox medicine has attempted to suppress the competition of healthy alternatives. The AMA long referred to chiropractic as an "unscientific cult," and held that it was unethical for medical doctors to associate with "unscientific practitioners." In 1987, a court opinion was issued proclaiming that the AMA had violated Section 1 of the Sherman Antitrust Act and had "engaged in an unlawful conspiracy in restraint of trade 'to contain and eliminate the chiropractic profession' (*Wilk v. American Medical Association*)." The court opinion further stated that the "AMA had entered into a long history of illegal behavior." A permanent injunction was issued against the AMA to prevent further illegal activities.[2] Both the U.S. Court of Appeals *and* the U.S. Supreme Court upheld the decision in 1990.[3] Dr. Chester Wilk and four (4) other chiropractors took on the AMA and won a victory, not only for the chiropractic profession, but for American citizens' freedom of choice in health care. The modus operandi of conventional medicine is to systematically attempt to suppress, disparage, and discredit any alternative challenge to their monopoly, often referring to alternative practitioners as "quacks." In fact, the AMA had established a McCarthyesque "Committee on Quackery" in 1963, with the primary mission of blacklisting the chiropractic profession.[4]

Similar to the chiropractic profession, alternative healing practitioners use natural methods to promote health and healing. This natural approach runs counter to the surgical and pharmaceutical approach promoted by orthodox medicine. Any alternative healing method is viewed as a competitive threat to the bottom line of Big Pharma, and must be eliminated at any cost and through whatever means possible.

The suppression of the right to choose our own health care is Un-American. It is Un-American to proliferate misinformation and to suppress information about beneficial alternatives to treating disease. The cancer cartel, as it exists today, is Un-American.

Boycott the pharmaceuticals. Insist upon vitamins and supplements that are chemical-free. Big Pharma cannot improve on nature. Chemicals are not the way to wellness. Natural is better. This is the way to wellness.

---

[1] Carrie Louise Daenell ND, "Resveratrol on 60 Minutes." <http://www.self growth.com/articles/Resveratrol_on_60_Minutes.html>.

[2] Wikipedia, <http://www.wikipedia.org>.

[3] "Chiropractic History-AMA v. Chiropractic," http://www.svpvril.com/ amavchir. html>.

[4] "American Medical Association," http://www.encognitive.com/node/1209>.

Friday, February 26, 2010

24. Wake-Up Call: The FDA Is NOT Your Friend

E-mails to my siblings . . .

—Original Message—

From: mbermel
Date: Friday, February 26, 2010, 8:15 p.m.
Subject: Brain Health, Macular degeneration, Parkinson's, Alzheimer's
           and Patient Rights
To: patty, mick, nina

I am reading a book called **FDA: Failure, Deception, Abuse: The Story of an Out-of-Control Government Agency and What it Means for your Health**. *The book talks about dementia, and how Phosphatidylserine (PS,) which is an essential brain nutrient, is effective for dementia. This supplement was introduced in 1988, and the FDA fought to keep it off the market despite clear benefits for elderly Americans. Finally in 2003, the FDA after a legal battle, permitted statements on the labels of PS bottles saying that PS may reduce the risk of cognitive dysfunction in the elderly, and it may reduce the risk of dementia.[1] Google it, you can buy it on the Life Extension website (lef.org). Read the book too; it is a revelation. The FDA is not just a bunch of mindless bureaucrats; this agency is pure, orchestrated evil.*

The book states that "Thalidomide has been shown to halt the proliferation of blood vessels, an effect that may help starve certain cancers and protect against blindness induced by wet macular degeneration." Because thalidomide can also halt limb development in pregnancy, this drug has been banned by the FDA except for treatment of complications related to leprosy (this covers about 50 Americans per year). This drug cannot be prescribed for cancer or macular degeneration, even though this drug has been shown to be effective.[2] Who is the FDA protecting? A person who has cancer or macular degeneration should have the RIGHT TO CHOOSE. But they don't, because of FDA suppression. From the same essay: "Neurogenerative diseases such as Alzheimer's have no effective treatment. A drug called memantine may delay the progression of Alzheimer's and Parkinson's Diseases. Memantine works by a different mechanism than current FDA-approved drugs such as Aricept and Tacrine. Memantine has been used in Germany for the last ten years, but it remains bogged down in FDA-mandated clinical trials. Four million American Alzheimer's disease patients anxiously await."[3]

Could our parents have been helped with their Parkinson's Disease, macular degeneration, dementia, Alzheimer's disease? You decide. What lies in *our* future? The time to fix this travesty is *now*. We need to wake up to the fact that the FDA is not our friend. The FDA is not about truth or health. It will not guide you on your way to wellness.

[1,2,3] Life Extension Foundation, *FDA: Failure, Deception, Abuse: The Story of an Out-of-Control Government Agency and What it Means for your Health* (Mount Jackson, VA: Praktikos Books, 2010).

Tuesday, March 2, 2010

25. The Gift of Cancer

Cancer is a gift to be embraced and then let go. It has no hold on my life. It entered my life briefly and had the effect of a huge red stop sign.

Everything in my life came suddenly screeching to a halt. This thing had to be dealt with. How? It was unclear.

I am a first-degree black belt in the art of Shaolin Kempo Karate. A fearless warrior in search of truth. I set about preparing for my ultimate test. I prepared mentally, spiritually, psychologically, and physically. As soon as I could move, I began my qi gong exercises, strengthening every day my mind, body, spirit. I pushed past my limits every day. A gift? This requires explanation. Of course, this is not a gift in the traditional sense. And there were moments of sheer terror, fear, and unbelievable stress. But a gift, nonetheless.

At a meditation group last night, I drew three cards: *Friendships, Intention,* and *Emergence.* The greater explanation of each:

> *Friendships* are changing and new friendships are developing based upon common understandings, but old and new friendships are all based in love. During this time of recovery and renaissance, I am experiencing a tremendous outpouring of love from friends and family. *This is a wonderful gift.*
>
> *Intention* must be set to discover the true purpose and meaning of life. Robust health must be chosen; the intention must be set. Once established, then there is the freedom to choose my life's path unfettered by outside influences. *This is a wonderful gift.*
>
> *Emergence* of peace and happiness and the expression of true inner self support the fearless pursuit of my life choices. *This is a wonderful gift.*

Without the presentation of cancer, these gifts would not have been presented. Now that this disease has brought its gifts and its lessons, I have embraced it, expressed gratitude, and let it go.

I am moving steadfastly on my true path, with my strengthened spirit, and the love of my husband, family, and friends, and I have left cancer behind. The storm is behind; sunny skies lie ahead. This is my truth and inspiration, my way to wellness.

Thursday, March 4, 2010

26. The Chemo Patient Dies of Chemo, Not of Cancer

My sister told me today that her co-worker's wife died. The wife had brain cancer, and the husband believes that it was the chemotherapy that killed her.

The thing that I learned about chemo is that it is more about the money than about saving lives. The cancer industry is *not* an altruistic enterprise. An enterprise yes, but not an altruistic one. It is the Ponzi scheme of the medical profession in the sense that even if "they" wanted to stop bilking people of their savings and their lives, to do so would expose the fraud. "They" cannot stop. I believe that Bernie Madoff was quoted as saying that he wanted to stop, but that he couldn't. The same principle (or lack of it) applies in this situation. How do you come clean? They must continue to perpetrate the fraud by perpetuating the lies. They cannot stop. They cannot admit that they were wrong *now* because to do so would be admitting their responsibility for the millions of lives that were sacrificed at the altar of their greed. The madness must stop. My sister's co-worker was right; the chemotherapy killed his wife.

Just say no to chemo. It is *not* truth; it is *not* the way to wellness.

Thursday, March 4, 2010

27. Waiting for You to Die . . .

When a diagnosis of this magnitude is received, some very subtle changes occur in others' perceptions of you. They expect you to die, and they are genuinely surprised when you don't. Friends will call and say that they thought they had better check to see how you are doing. I call these the "checking to see if you're still alive" calls. They ask how you are. If you reply, "OK," or "good," then the response is "well, hang in there." So you must elevate the response to the superlative: "great!" "How are you?" "Great!" "Really?" "Yes, *really*!" "Really, you're feeling OK?" "Yes, I am feeling *great*!" This does not happen during normal social interactions. This happens only after a cancer diagnosis.

People *are* waiting for you to die . . . and then you don't. They are not consciously standing on the sidelines, cheering you on to cross the finish line to death, but they are subconsciously waiting for your mortality to manifest. Believing in alternative medicine, good medicine, requires a leap of faith. We have been brainwashed into believing in traditional medicine, which, in the case of cancer treatment, is *bad* medicine. We have to consciously abandon a deeply entrenched belief system which is based upon nothing more than continual media repetition. If the belief in chemotherapy is challenged, the person questioned initially reacts as if hearing blasphemy, as if something sacrosanct has been attacked. However, the person questioned has absolutely no data to substantiate their belief. This can readily be tested by conducting your own random survey, and asking the questions, "1) Do you believe that chemotherapy is effective in treating cancer, and 2) if so, why?" The first question will generally be answered "Yes," but the second question seems to stump people. They cannot explain *why* they believe that chemotherapy is effective. If you don't know why you believe that something is effective, you should explore it fully before you agree to it. Don't just agree to it because you think you have no choice. You, like everyone else, have been brainwashed. You *do* have a choice.

Although your family, friends, neighbors, and co-workers do not consciously want you to die, your death will validate their belief system, and they can rationalize, "I warned her to listen to the doctors, but she didn't, and now she's dead." However, staying alive proves the point and makes the case for alternative, beneficial, "good" medicine. With each passing day, week, month, and year of your life, your circle of friends discovers the truth that chemo is not the way to wellness by simple observation: you are still alive.

Perception. Self-awareness. These elements are critical to health recovery. When someone accepts the poison of chemotherapy, the toxin causes their hair to fall out. They are immediately identified as a cancer patient. But they are actually a chemo patient. When they look in people's eyes, what they see is pity because people know that they will die. People start to distance themselves from the chemo patient; they are preparing for the inevitable loss, the death, the grief. Hair loss is a visual indicator that the chemo patient's body is toxic and out of balance. People expect that you will die because likely you will.

This is the difference between cancer and chemo. Chemo kills; cancer does not have to. It is a manageable disease. Choose "healthy living" over toxic treatments, and when you look in people's eyes, you will see normalcy, not sympathy.

I really enjoy meeting new people now, because I don't mention my recent health issue, and they treat me as if I am as normal and healthy as anyone else. And so I am.

Perception. Self-awareness. This is huge in the recovery process. Think of yourself as being robustly healthy. Then others will too. *And you will be robustly healthy.*

This is the way to wellness.

Friday, March 19, 2010

28. "It's Better in the Bahamas"

A vacation to the Bahamas took on special significance as a symbolic turning point in my recovery process. Four (4) months ago, I could only imagine myself on an island beach in the Caribbean. Had I blindly and obediently followed medical recommendation, I would certainly be lying in my bed, bald, weak, and ravaged by toxic "medicine." In order to escape the terrible reality of that scenario, my experience of an island beach in the Caribbean would still be confined to the limits of my imagination.

On this day, I am grateful for my robust health. My energy level is very high, my mental outlook is very positive. I have returned to my life as it was before this crisis of health, but I have returned a stronger person, a better person, and a more appreciative person. This has been a game-changer. Life is good. And I am grateful.

My path to excellent health has taken me to my island paradise. I find my inspiration in the beauty that surrounds us, and in my renewed ability to appreciate that beauty. I think of Mary Yevchak, whose path led her to Freeport, Bahamas. She went to this island paradise to fight her cancer and escape the U.S. cancer establishment in April-May 1984. In May 1984, I was in Freeport, Bahamas on my honeymoon. Little did I know that at the same time, Mary Yevchak was there fighting for her life and fighting for truth, a battle that I would join years later. I think of her bravery in testifying at a Congressional hearing, in trail-blazing in this disease, in fighting the cancer industry and resisting the "standard of care" treatments, in fighting for the rights of patients to choose their own treatments.

Truly, "It's better in the Bahamas." This is truth *and* inspiration.

Friday, March 19, 2010

29. The Unheralded Parsley Sprig

I learned from reading John Irving's new book *Last Night at Twisted River* that parsley is pure chlorophyll.[1] So now I am adding chopped parsley to everything! It is not the wimpy garnish that everyone ignores and leaves on the plate. Parsley, according to Dr. Gillian McKeith is "the culinary multi-vitamin, a nutrient powerhouse," containing essential fatty acids, vitamins, and nutrients, supporting organ function and stimulating the immune system; it contains chlorophyll, which inhibits the "bad" bacteria in the body.[2]

Why didn't I learn all these things before the age of 56 1/2? Why did I think as a child that bacon toast was a good breakfast? And spam a good lunch? And Texas Wieners a good dinner? It is not surprising that health issues manifested. But I was a child in the '50s and '60s, when people were cost-conscious and not health-conscious.

Then people became health conscious. But the trend toward better health and better eating was thwarted by the food industry. The food industry decided to join with the chemical industry and create foods in the lab. They decided to produce food cheaply, to add high fructose corn syrup to virtually every processed food item on the shelf, including ketchup! Deciphering the labels on food packages literally requires a chemical engineering background. We do not know what we are eating, but we do know that we are eating chemicals. The chemicals that we ingest start the disease time bomb ticking. When (not if) the disease manifests, we move down the assembly line and we are turned over to the pharmaceutical industry, which attempts to "treat" us with chemicals, albeit different chemicals than those that made us sick in the first place.

Parsley, a pure, simple, natural sprig that lines the way to wellness.

---

[1] John Irving, Last Night at Twisted River (New York: Random House, 2009).

[2] Dr. Gillian McKeith, Living Food for Health: 12 Natural Superfoods to Transform your Health (London: Piatkus Books, 2000).

Saturday, March 27, 2010

30. "I'm as mad as hell . . ."

In 1976, a movie called *Network* produced a memorable quote that is still relevant over thirty years later. *Network* was written by Paddy Chayefsky, and the part of Howard Beale was played by Peter Finch. The scene went like this:

Howard Beale: I don't have to tell you things are bad. Everybody knows things are bad. We know the air is unfit to breathe and our food is unfit to eat, and we sit watching our TV's . . . as if that's the way it's supposed to be. We know things are bad—worse than bad. They're crazy. It's like everything everywhere is going crazy, so we don't go out anymore. We sit in the house, and slowly the world we are living in is getting smaller, and all we say is, 'Please, at least leave us alone in our living rooms. Let me have my toaster and my TV and my steel-belted radials and I won't say anything. Just leave us alone.' Well, I'm not gonna leave you alone. I want you to get mad! I don't want you to protest. I don't want you to riot—I don't want you to write to your congressman because I wouldn't know what to tell you to write. All I know is that first you've got to get mad.

Howard Beale: [*shouting*] You've got to say, 'I'm a HUMAN BEING, Goddamnit! My life has VALUE!' So I want you to get up now. I want all of you to get up out of your chairs. I want you to get up right now and go to the window. Open it, and stick your head out, and yell,

[*shouting*]

Howard Beale: 'I'M AS MAD AS HELL, AND I'M NOT GOING TO TAKE THIS ANYMORE!' I want you to get up right now, sit up, go to your windows, open them and stick your head out and yell—'I'm as mad as hell and I'm not going to take this anymore!' Things have got to change. But first, you've gotta get mad! You've got to say, 'I'm as mad as hell, and I'm not going to take this anymore!' Then we'll figure out what to do . . . But first get up out of your chairs, open the window, stick your head out, and yell, and say it:

Howard Beale: [*screaming at the top of his lungs*] "I'M AS MAD AS HELL, AND I'M NOT GOING TO TAKE THIS ANYMORE!" [1]

In 1979, I spent some summer weekends on Fire Island, during one of which I met my husband. One of the weekend houseguests was undergoing chemotherapy treatment for cancer. Bob was the first chemotherapy patient I had ever met, and I was struck by his diminishing physical energy. With every ensuing weekend, he became progressively weaker. One weekend, Fire Island experienced a loss of electricity, and there was no communication from the (then) Long Island Lighting Company (LILCO) as to when power would be restored. Bob organized a group of "house people," got them to get out of their houses, go to the dock, face the mainland of Long Island, and yell at the top of their lungs:

I'M AS MAD AS HELL, AND I'M NOT GOING TO TAKE THIS ANYMORE!"

Viscerally, we knew that this was a cathartic act for Bob, yet we all supported him, knowing full well that LILCO would never hear this protest from across the Great South Bay. Bob's displaced rage was not at the loss of electricity, but at the impending loss of his life. Bob died in the fall of 1979, ostensibly from cancer, but in actuality from the toxic treatment his body could not take anymore.

I was young and couldn't understand: if he was being treated, why did he die? Wasn't the treatment supposed to make him better? Why didn't it work? Why did he endure the pain and suffering of the treatment just to die in the end? There were many questions, but no answers. Even now, many deaths later, death is accepted as the expected outcome of cancer. If someone survives, the remark is "wow, they were one of the lucky ones," or "they got it early." Sometimes when I tell people that I had ovarian cancer, the initial look is one of disbelief. They cannot believe this because, first, I am alive, and second, I look robustly healthy. When someone inevitably dies after doing "everything possible" which is a euphemism for surgery, chemo, and radiation (cut, poison, and burn), the platitudes are abundant: "they fought the good fight," "they did everything possible," or "it was just too late." This is all—what's another word for bullshit? Bullshit. We must tell it as it is. We must stop accepting death as the expected outcome of a cancer diagnosis. That is unacceptable. Cancer is a manageable disease.

Since President Nixon declared war on cancer in 1971, not too much has changed in conventional treatment. There has been very little progress and everyone just accepts that, continuing to believe the blithe assurances of the American Cancer Society that "the cure is just around the corner."[2] This is *not acceptable*. We all need to be inspired by Bob, and rise up and shout: **I'M AS MAD AS HELL, AND I'M NOT GOING TO TAKE THIS ANYMORE!"** This is pure inspiration. It is the way to wellness.

Do not get mad about getting cancer; get mad about the lies in cancer treatment.

Just say no to chemo. Chemo is not truth. It is *not* the way to wellness.

---

[1] "Memorable Quotes for 'Network'," <http://www.imdb.com/title /tt0074958/ quotes>.

[2] *Healing Cancer from the Inside Out*, dir. Mike Anderson, DVD, 2008).

Wednesday, March 31, 2010

31. The Right of Survivorship

The right of survivorship is generally defined in estate law as the division of real property among the remaining survivors upon the death of one of the principals.

I like to think of the right of survivorship as the right of a person to survive an ordeal. Every person has that right, and every person must believe in that right. Fear cannot be given a toehold in this process. After being told by too many oncologists that my life was limited, my inner voice became a whisper, very close to being extinguished by fear. Somehow, I still managed to hear that weak, little inner voice calling out "don't believe them." And now that inner voice is bellowing to others in the same predicament: **"DON'T BELIEVE THEM!!!"**

The right of survivorship is predicated upon several conditions: 1) no matter how dire, the situation must be survivable, and most situations are; 2) the person must want to survive; 3) accurate information must be accessed; 4) correct decisions must be made based on fact and truth; 5) facilities with the word "cancer" in the name must be avoided, choosing instead a facility that focuses on "wellness" and not on the disease; 6) there must be present an element of luck, karma, faith, divine intervention, and inspiration.

I fought hard for my right of survivorship, and my survival continues to depend upon these ideal conditions. I share with others this instruction manual on how to survive cancer. We have the right to survive. In order to survive, we have the right to expect freedom of information and freedom of choice. This war on cancer is now about our rights and our freedoms.

I am a survivor, not *because* of chemotherapy, but because I *avoided* it. This is truth. This is my way to wellness.

Saturday, April 3, 2010

32. Profile of a Chi Gung Student

In 1993, my house was burglarized. Aside from the loss of jewelry having great sentimental value, there was also the trauma of the intrusion, as my sense of security in my own home was shaken. The psychological effect played on my mind: what would have happened if I was home at the time, and unable to defend myself? I decided to take action: we installed an alarm system, we adopted a black Labrador Retriever, and I enrolled in a self-defense course.

The alarm system helped to restore my sense of security, Roxanne became a wonderful friend who defended the house from any crows entering the yard, and the self-defense course resulted in a first-degree black belt in Shaolin Kempo Karate nine years later.

During that same time period, I also developed an interest in energy work through Healing Touch. I spent several weekends taking courses and I became a Level 2 Healing Touch practitioner.

I spent one winter learning the long form of T'ai Chi. I loved the flow of energy. Between Karate, Healing Touch, and T'ai Chi, I was tapping into the energy field previously unknown to me. I was hooked on chi.

As an adjunct to my Karate training, I bought a book called *Introduction to Chi Gung*, and I followed the illustrations and descriptions to learn the beginning elements of breathing and movement. This was my first introduction to qi gong.

As I moved through the aging process, I was finding the intensity of karate grueling and punishing, and I began to think that I needed to step down. I was searching. I was not a marathoner like brothers Jack and Mick, but I had always been physically active. I was a 10k runner at a 7-minute pace, a skier, a golfer. But I needed to tap into the *chi*. I tried Curves and found it too repetitive and boring. I tried yoga. I tried Pilates. I took a 4-week T'ai Chi course. I bought a DVD called *Qigong Beginning Practice*[1] and followed along with the movements. I remembered that I had attended a 1-night library class in qi gong, and I remembered that I somewhat enjoyed it. I searched online for the information on the school, and I corresponded with the Laoshi by e-mail. I decided to give it a try.

In October 2009, I underwent extensive surgery and came out with a diagnosis of stage 1a ovarian cancer. While in the hospital, still unable to walk, I began breathing exercises and simple qi gong arm movements. At home, I continued these motions every morning. I pushed beyond my limits every day, moving from sitting to standing to walking postures. I researched extensively and found *Guo Lin Chi Gong* online and watched that website's video, *Fighting Cancer with Your Body's Internal Energy*.[2] I memorized the walking Chi Gong movements and went outside to my backyard, asking my husband to watch me in case I fell over. The movement begins with gathering positive healing energy from the sky, from the living beings on the earth, and finally from the earth itself: tapping into the universal chi. Every morning without fail, I go outside and connect with this energy and practice qi gong outside, stopped only by blizzard conditions.

How did disease enter my life? I am physically active. I eat healthy foods, avoiding processed foods, high fructose corn syrup, artificial sweeteners. What was the cause? In retrospect, my chi was disturbed, I was not committed to life, my system was in a state of imbalance. I had a series of losses in my life, moving from one loss to the next, connected by periods of grief. My sister-in-law Mary. My cat Saucy. His brother Tigger. My brother Jack. My brother-in-law Peter. My dear friend Taylor. My Roxanne. My mother-in-law Virginia. The grief kept accumulating. I abandoned the healing energy work, blaming myself for not being able to heal the people and animals I loved.

Qi gong has helped to restore balance to my body, mind, spirit. "Turn, look, and leave behind." As Laoshi said, "Let go of whatever does not serve me." I have let it all go. I have found my core again, my chi flows freely, I am happy and healthy. The sadness is gone. I am committed to life.

I came into the kwoon with an open mind and no expectations. My biggest challenge is adjusting to the noncombativeness and peacefulness of qi gong, as well as to the slower pace, as compared to karate. Sometimes when I step onto the mat, I step back in time to the dojo, expecting to have to defend myself against attackers with a "crane's wing" or a "snake bite." The biggest benefit of qi gong is the restoration of my health. The path to my recovery is "healthy living" in mind, body, and spirit. Exercise is essential, and qi gong is the foundation that makes all other exercise possible. I skied on Valentine's Day. I golfed in March. With qi gong, all things are possible.

The qi gong school is an unexpected gift. I found that I have entered into a peaceful, supportive place, surrounded by Reiki practitioners, kind and caring people, a very thoughtful and mindful Laoshi, a haven where universal chi flows freely.

In Chinese philosophy, the "Tao" is the way or the path. Life is good, and when faced with death, I chose life. My intention is to stay for a while longer. Through Chi Gung, I have found the Tao; I have found truth, inspiration, my way to wellness.

---

1   *Qigong Beginning Practice with Francesco Garripoli & Daisy Lee-Garripoli*. Dir. Michael Badertscher. DVD. Gaiam, Inc., 2004.

2   "Guolin Qi Gong-Cancer Buster. Walking Qi Gong." <http://www.qigong chinesehealth.com/walking_qigong>

Sunday, April 11, 2010

33. A World without Cancer

Last year I met Ruth on the golf course at the local country club where I am a member. We hit it off, and we try to play regularly on Sunday afternoons. After a long and particularly brutal winter, I was anxious to play again. And so we started playing again, Ruth and I, on Sunday afternoons. I was apprehensive: this was a test of my physical capacity and stamina. Will I be able to play after everything that I have been through?

Ruth is a Christian Scientist. The belief system of a Christian Scientist does not include belief in cancer, or in any disease for that matter. "We are spirit, not matter," I learned from Ruth. In the world according to Ruth, cancer simply does not exist. When I play golf with Ruth, I am playing with someone who does not acknowledge that I was ever ill, someone who believes that I never had cancer because, very simply, cancer does not exist.

Ruth believes that all things are possible, and that we should have an "expectancy of good." When I play golf with Ruth, I hit great shots beyond myself, but more importantly, I play with strength and prowess. I play as if I am in perfect health, because I am. I am living, for a time, in Ruth's world, a world without cancer. I take this thinking home with me, and make it my world as well. The desire to live in a world without cancer can be realized, if only we believe. Find truth. Be inspired. This is the way to wellness.

Wednesday, April 21, 2010

34. *Australia*

A friend recently told me that she had a mole that had to be biopsied. It turned out to be benign, but when she heard the word "biopsy," she was struck with fear, unable to think or talk or even breathe.

In a scene from the movie *Australia*, Nullah (the aboriginal boy) stared death in the eye and conquered his fear, as the thundering herd of bulls approached him. He was heroically trying to stop the herd from stampeding over the edge of the cliff. He believed that if you stood and looked the bull in the eye, the bull would stop. So he stood his ground at the edge of the cliff, and sang his brave little song to stop the bulls, and as they approached, he quivered with fear, yet stood bravely, looked the lead bull in the eye to make him stop, and wondrously, the herd literally stopped in its tracks, yards from Nullah and the edge of the cliff. Nullah collapsed in relief; the danger had passed. He was safe.[1]

When cancer approaches, it is best to stand bravely and stare it down. Look it squarely in the eye. It will stop. Don't let it paralyze you with fear. Rise above it and take action. You will overcome it in your own way. Become the fearless warrior in search of truth. Say the word "cancer" over and over again in your mind until it loses its power over you. Find your way. Believe. You are safe. You are on the way to wellness.

---

[1]   *Australia*, dir. Baz Luhrmann, DVD, Bazmark Films, 2008.

Sunday, April 25, 2010

35. The Bogus War on Cancer

In 1971, President Richard Nixon declared war on cancer with the signing of the National Cancer Act. He compared curing cancer with going to the moon.[1]

In this "war," where is the battlefield? Where is the commander-in-chief? Where are the generals? Where is the battle plan? Who are the combatants? Why hasn't the artillery changed in almost forty years? Why are we still accepting collateral damage? Why are the victims of this war the innocent civilians? Where are the antiwar protestors? Why aren't we winning this war? When will we learn that "wars" declared on diseases (like cancer) and social issues (like poverty, drugs, litter) cannot be won?

The war on cancer is bogus; it is a farce. It has devolved to a situation of "every man for himself" in hand-to-hand combat. Do not let yourself get drafted into this war. It is the medical equivalent of another Vietnam, another Iraq. This war cannot be won.

In almost forty years, the only outcome of this "war" is the stark reality that we can do better. There has been no victory. Researchers have had the time and the money to solve this problem, to actually cure cancer. Yes, cure. It should be no more complicated than setting a broken leg. Broken leg? No problem. Cancer? No problem. Going to the moon? No problem. But cancer? "Houston, we have a problem." Big Pharma is making too much money to want to find the cure. The miles logged in for "walk for the cure" events are at least equivalent to the 238,857 miles to the moon. People are walking in the wrong direction. *Stop* "walking for the cure." Stage a sit-down protest; this was the action that made a difference in 1971. We sat down and demanded that the war in Vietnam end. Sit down now and demand that the *real* cure for cancer be found, that the beneficial treatments be released from suppression, that the toxic ineffective chemotherapy be ended. The charade must stop. Let people know that sometimes the best action is no action. It is better to focus on making the effort to improve health through nutrition and exercise. Medication is not the solution to everything. Sometimes medication makes the situation worse. Demand that the FDA work with researchers who are on the right path to a real cure, instead of supporting Big Pharma with their bogus treatments. Demand that the FDA stop their gestapo tactics of harassing those practitioners whose treatments actually help. We need to find the cause. Without focusing on the cause, we are being set up for future disaster. Without getting to the root cause, it will come back. Similar to applying a toxic weed killer to weeds, surrounding flowers will be damaged, even killed. However, without destroying the root of the weed, the weed will return, more virulent than ever. We need to identify the cause, we need to identify the solution.

A friend recently diagnosed with carcinoma remarked that it was surprising how little the doctors know about the cause of the disease, and how little they know about the treatment for the disease.

Almost 600,000 Americans die every year from cancer and/or cancer treatments. How are these deaths justified? They are *not* justified. They are *not* necessary. We deserve better. Demand it. END THE BOGUS WAR ON CANCER. It is not truth. It is not inspiration. It is *not* the way to wellness.

---

[1] <http://www.dtp.nci.nih.gov/timeline/noflash/milestones/M4_Nixon.htm>.

Thursday, April 29, 2010

36. The Survivor Bowl

Mick is a world traveler, having spent most of his adult life as an "expatriate" living in various resurgent countries, none of which would be featured any time soon in Condé Nast. From his recent trip to Rwanda, he presented me with a vibrant red hand-woven bowl with the design of a star worked into the base. These bowls are generically referred to as Rwanda Peace Baskets, and are crafted as part of the "Path to Peace" project. This bowl was likely created by one of the women who survived the horrific genocide of 1994, when the Hutu hunted down and massacred 800,000 Tutsi and moderate Hutu in 100 days, and the world viewed this atrocity with a blind eye. The artisan community characterizes their hand crafts as "symbolizing insight and sustenance through human effort." I call mine the "Survivor Bowl," and it is now one of my prized possessions; it symbolizes the bravery of these women, these people who survived the unthinkable. It raises the state of survivorship to a new level. I have been referred to as a "survivor" of a disease. My struggle, my courage, and my will to live pales in comparison to the struggles, the courage, and the will to live of these survivors. From the survivorship of these people emerged a creative life force that produces beautiful and useful pieces of art. The inspiration of this Survivor Bowl will be a daily reminder to me that there are many people in this world who have survived far worse ordeals than mine, and from the darkness, they emerged as brilliant, shining stars. Be inspired by those who survived horrific trials by standing strong. Find the truth; confront the lies. This is pure inspiration. This is the "path to peace," the way to wellness.

Friday, April 30, 2010

37. "Everybody Loves a Winner"

. . . is a song written by Jerry Garcia and performed live by the Levon Helm Band at a concert for which my brother Mick and I had front row seats, and the great privilege of watching this almost seventy-year-old artist perform with purity of heart and soul. Music is the great healer. It taps into the inner recesses of the soul and brings out the positive healing energy. Everybody loves a winner. It is human nature. People do not like to be close to others who are losers. In a physical state, this means that if people are in a situation where their health is compromised, others previously close to them will start to emotionally distance themselves so as to, first of all, not suffer greatly when the seemingly inevitable occurs, and secondly, so as not to be reminded of their own mortality and frailties. People are uncomfortable with other people being suspended between life and death. But everybody loves a winner. Like Levon. Who at the beginning of the century faced throat cancer. And survived. And thrived. Why? Because of his choice to live; because of the music. In his own words, "I'm back, and I've still got music to share." The crowd loved him, yelling out repeatedly and unabashedly, "We love you Levon!" Everybody loves a winner. And as he finally left the stage after a rare encore to a standing ovation, he touched his heart with his hand and offered it to the crowd, saying "I love you too." A wrenching separation. And from the front row, one could see into the wings of the stage where a roadie gently covered this aging musician's shoulders with a blanket. Levon, the blues master. Levon, the survivor. The show was over. Until tomorrow comes.

"Everybody loves a winner." Truth. Pure inspiration. The way to wellness.

Friday, April 30, 2010

38. Watch Your Supplements: The Big Pharma Shell Game

Big Pharma is working through our elected federal representatives to eliminate supplements, which represents the only competitive force that interferes with their profit-making ability. Any natural supplement that is effective will be replicated chemically so that Big Pharma can profit.

Pharmaceutical lobbying + Federal legislation = Loss of Supplements.

Big Pharma uses their obscene profits to lobby our representatives, which means wining and dining them and convincing them to represent not *us*—"we the People," but *them*—'we the Pharma.'

This is a shell game that Big Pharma is playing. Keep your eye on the legislation. Your supplements may disappear underneath it.

———————

—Original Message—

From: Life Extension
Date: Friday, April 30, 2010, 1:19 a.m.
Subject: Yet Another Threat to Supplements on Capitol Hill
To: mbermel

"Life Extension Foundation®

Yet Another Threat to Supplements on Capitol Hill

The threat of a regulatory stranglehold over dietary supplements has intensified.

Earlier this year, Sen. John McCain introduced a bill that would have given the FDA draconian new powers. A citizen's revolt ensued that caused that bill to be sidelined. We are being watchful that Sen. McCain does not try to slip some of his oppressive original proposals into another Senate bill.

The urgent issue we face today is language Rep. Henry Waxman snuck into the already passed Wall Street Reform Bill (H.R. 4173) that he hopes to get into the Senate bill. This language would give unelected FTC bureaucrats arbitrary authority to impose crippling requirements that will drive up the costs of supplements or remove them from the market entirely.

It is imperative that consumers e-mail their Senators to keep this language out of the Senate version of the Wall Street Reform Bill and out of any later version voted on by the House and Senate.

What Is Really Going On Here

Pharmaceutical companies recognize that their greatest competitive threat comes from low-cost dietary supplements that are virtually free of side effects. The most efficient way to destroy this competition is to have Congress enact legislation that will enable federal agencies to eradicate consumer access to dietary supplements.

To give you an idea of how much money is involved, just look at the cost of prescription drug fish oil sold under the trade name Lovaza®. A 30-day supply of Lovaza® sells for around $195.00. Consumers can obtain the same quantity of EPA/DHA fish oil for under $32.00 as a dietary supplement. With the passage of the Medicare Prescription Drug Act and Health Care Reform Act, the federal government (that means you) pays outrageously inflated prices for fish oil prescriptions and other drugs.

The pharmaceutical industry heavily lobbied Congress to obligate Medicare to shell out full retail price for prescription drugs. In the case of prescription fish oil, taxpayers pay 500% more than what consumers pay for the same amount of fish oil as a dietary supplement.

Pharmaceutical companies now want to erect so many new restrictions over dietary supplements that consumers (and taxpayers) will be forced to pay outlandish prescription drug prices for fish oil and other low-cost nutrients. As most of you know, taxes will soon be raised and new government debt created to fund these lavish subsidies to drug companies. It is this kind of institutional corruption that bankrupts governments around the world. We fear that citizen apathy may enable this corrupt legislation to be enacted into law, which will hasten Medicare's date with insolvency, while saddling consumers with higher dietary supplement prices, if the supplements are available at all. If this legislation is passed, our fear is that many supplements will disappear or that Americans will be unable to afford their supplements and will succumb to a host of deficiency-related diseases."

Lovaza is marketed in television advertisements by Glaxo Smith Klein (GSK) as "the prescription that starts in the sea," "where nature meets science."[1] This is big business. If you can't eliminate the competition, use any means to take it over. According to the official website[2], Lovaza is different from dietary supplements, in that "supplements are not FDA-approved to treat a specific disease . . ." According to the TV ad, Lovaza is "Omega-3-acid ethyl esters" and is "the only Omega 3 *medication* that's FDA-approved. You can't get it at a health food store. Side effects may include burping, infection, flu-like symptoms, upset stomach, and change in sense of taste. Ask your doctor about Lovaza." Big Pharma is starting to respond to the challenge of natural supplements. The FDA can only hold off public demand for natural supplements for so long. GSK has the vision to see a niche market, and is setting out to carve out its share. Pharma Fish Oil now. Pharma Resveratrol soon. What is the next Pharma-supplement? Watch your supplements: Big Pharma is trying to abscond with them. Demand the right to choose the natural way to wellness.

---

[1]   Lovaza television advertisement.

[2]   "Lovaza," <http://www.lovaza.com>.

Monday, May 3, 2010

39. Another Casualty of the War on Cancer

My friend Loretta e-mailed today. Her father had been to the emergency room twice over the weekend and his liver was shutting down. He was diagnosed in the fall with stage IV colon cancer, and approached his disease as something that he would overcome. He had a fighting spirit. He did everything the doctors told him to do. He was a good patient, unlike me. Not difficult, unlike me. Not questioning, unlike me. Did that make the difference? Possibly. I said no to chemo; he said yes. I physically shudder to think that I could have been in his shoes, facing certain death with the reality of failing organs.

How is it that the oncological profession can still daily convince people to willingly go to their deaths? By mouthing the words, "standard of care." These are soothing words. "Standard." "Care." How can that be harmful? "Standard of care" is a euphemism for "we don't know what else to do." Be very wary if you hear those words uttered.

When people are told that, with chemo, they will have six (6) months to a year to live, that means that the chemo will, in fact, kill them in six (6) months to a year. That much is known. When they say that you will die in less than a year, they don't mean that chemo is the treatment that is going to cure your disease, and that if you are strong enough, you will survive it. They mean what they say: you *will* die. Believe it. Find a treatment that won't kill you. Chemo is toxic, and it takes about six (6) months to a year to sufficiently cause enough internal damage to slowly kill the body. The spirit slowly dies as well. A spirit that started off strong and determined to survive, gradually gives in to the ravages of the toxins on the body, and gives up the battle. Chemo is too strong an opponent. You can't conquer chemo. And when the bad medicine fails, the surviving family and friends have already been trained to blame the patient: he waited too long to go to the doctor, she gave up hope, he smoked for too many years, she didn't complete her chemo treatments. We search for some reason why the treatment failed; there must be *something* that the person did or didn't do that resulted in their death. The truth is this: chemo is just bad medicine that just does not work.

Chemotherapy causes a slow, painful death. At least with a Kevorkian treatment, patients knew the truth and made an informed choice, and their choice was death. They knew exactly what they were signing up for. And they died quickly and painlessly.

With chemotherapy, patients are not told the truth, they are not given truthful information to make an informed choice; they do not know that they are choosing death. They are forced to take their medicine to the bitter end.

Friends have told me stories of their mothers and fathers, dying in a cancer hospital, and still being administered the maximum sub-lethal dosage of chemotherapy. Some families protested and went "AMA" ("against medical advice"). Other families desperately accepted the treatment and the patient, who is at that point heavily sedated to handle the pain caused by chemotherapy, is subjected to yet even more chemotherapy in a last-ditch heroic yet futile effort to "beat the disease." In this way, the doctors can reassure the family that "they did everything possible," and the survivors can sleep at night.

The final stop for the patient is hospice care. This is where the patient, who is so beaten down by the ravages of chemotherapy, is taken to die. Although the word sounds very soothing, it is, like the rest of a misguided cancer odyssey, misleading. The patient rarely walks in on their own strength, but if they do, these are the final steps of their life, the final steps on the misguided path. They are brought here to live out their final days, they are starved to death, and the reality of their pain is obscured by morphine. They will not walk out, they will not leave alive. They will take their final breath in hospice, on "palliative care." Palliative care has very interesting definitions:

1. "To relieve symptoms of; to ameliorate.
2. To hide or disguise.
3. To cover or disguise the seriousness of a mistake, offense, etc., by excuses and apologies.
4. To lessen the severity of; to extenuate, moderate, qualify.
5. To placate or mollify."[1]

Through hospice, the cancer industry disguises the seriousness of the mistake of chemotherapy. The patient's symptoms are relieved through morphine. The family is supported by compassionate staff, offering understanding and pity.

Everyone is placated through the palliative care offered by hospice. The cancer industry, to the bitter end, covers up what they have inflicted upon this unsuspecting human being. Yet the severity of death by chemo cannot be extenuated, moderated, or qualified. There is no acceptable excuse. There is no acceptable apology.

When a chemotherapy patient dies, the obituary will invariably report that the deceased died after a long, courageous battle against cancer. This is not truth. The long, courageous battle has been against chemotherapy. The chemotherapy patient did not have a chance. An indomitable spirit is no match for the destructive power of chemotherapy.

The real war on cancer must be a pitched battle between the patient and the cancer industry. At stake are patients' rights for truthful and beneficial treatments which can help them to manage their disease in a non-toxic, non-harmful way. The troops need to be rallied to avoid more casualties on our side, to avoid the collateral damage inflicted on the patient, to avoid the "friendly fire." The deaths inflicted by chemotherapy must be stopped.

Another casualty of the war on cancer is about to be claimed, barring a true miracle. There are millions of chemo victims strewn about the killing fields of the war on cancer. After chemo, all that is left is prayer: prayer for a miracle, prayer for the dying, prayer for the dead.

Chemotherapy is *not* truth. This is *not* the way to wellness.

---

[1]   <http://www.wiktionary.org>.

Saturday, May 15, 2010

40. Killing the Wrong Cells

—Original Message—
From: mick
Date: Sunday, April 4, 2010, 4:15 a.m.
Subject: New Hope
To: mbermel

Greetings from Kigali. You need to run to the newsstand and pick up the April 2010 Scientific American Mind and read the article on Brain Cancer. It has data that supports your argument. You need to read this, but the key points to the argument follow:

- *Current cancer treatment is to remove as many tumor cells as possible. When possible, this means to first remove them surgically, and then typically follow that with chemo and radiation—with the belief that it is effective, but the cancer can recur, with resistance to treatment. (Sometimes radiation or chemotherapy is used to shrink the tumor before surgery).*
- *This is what actually happens. There are two types of cancerous cells. The first is non-regenerative. The second type is regenerative and only they can proliferate all the cancer cells. The regenerative cells are also known as stem cells—which are highly resistant to any cancer treatment, thanks to their regenerative properties, vs. the non-regenerative cancerous cells.*
- *The stem cells make up only 3% of the cells in any given tumor, but they are the ones you want to go after. Other than the bulk of the non-regenerative cells, which can create problems, the non-regenerative cells don't pose the threat that the stem cells do.*
- *Here are the problems. First, by the time that the tumor is noticed, the more deadly stem cells have often migrated through bundles of nerves called white matter tracts to other locations. So even if you cut out the cancer, it is possible that the process is beginning somewhere else. Second, although chemo and radiation can shrink 97% of the tumor, they have little to no effect on the deadlier stem cells. Therefore, chemo is likely less effective than even you suspect, according to the article.*
- *The article mentions systems biology as trying to address this. This is how systems biology works. First, it is interested in determining movement along the pathways or white matter tracts, to see where the cancer has traveled. Find the tumor and look for all the pathways out*

of that area and you will see where the stem cells go. The systems folks don't usually refer to cancer as locational, such as brain or pancreas, but as pathways cancer. Second, examine the cell to determine if it is cancerous. Third, poison that cell and only that cell to eliminate it, with virtually no collateral damage.

I hope that is useful. Mick

—Original Message—

From: mbermel
Date: Sunday, April 4, 2010, 6:59 a.m.
Subject: Re: New Hope
To: mick

Hi Mick,

Thanks for the summary of the article. I'll get a copy.
I am happy that the researchers are finally on the right trail. But there is a disconnect between researchers and practitioners. The mainstream practitioners I have encountered are holding steady to the lie of chemo. There were actually some things that I could have done before surgery to minimize any spread, which my mainstream surgeon did not advise me of. I learned of this after the fact. What I am doing now is making my system so strong & healthy that it creates a hostile environment for any rogue cells to survive. Thanks for the input. Margaret

In an article published in the Scientific American Mind[1], Dr. Gregory Foltz states that all along, oncologists have been targeting the wrong cells in the treatment of brain cancer (glioma). Dr. Foltz writes that not much progress has been made in the treatment of this disease over the past thirty-five years; however, researchers have now finally discovered the "missing link" to successful treatment. Current "standard of care" for this disease is surgery to "de-bulk" the tumor, followed by chemo and radiation. "But," states Dr. Foltz, "most cancers recur, sometimes years later, often having acquired resistance to treatment." He explains that cancer treatment was designed to kill rapidly growing cells—cancer cells. But researchers were mystified as to why most cancers inevitably recur after treatment. Recent studies, according to Dr. Foltz, indicate that "this dogma may be dramatically wrong—and in a way that explains the mystery of recurrence." The "missing link" is that only a small number of cells can cause the growth of cancer cells; this "regenerative minority," according to Dr. Foltz, are "cancer stem cells." These cancer stem cells are very similar in characteristic to normal stem cells, and that is why they resist standard treatment. One characteristic of cancer stem cells found in brain tumors is that they have on their surface the same protein (CD133) that is found on the surface of "normal" neural stem cells. Standard treatment attacks fast-growing cells; these cancer stem cells are *not* fast-growing cells. The word Dr. Foltz uses is "quiescent"; they don't attract a lot of attention as they quietly lie in wait: "a cellular time bomb," Dr. Foltz terms them. The discovery of the properties of cancer stem cells is the "missing link" that, as Dr. Foltz explains, is the reason why "standard cancer treatments so often fail: those therapies target the wrong cells."

Dr. Foltz explains that the *properties* of cancer stem cells cause resistance to standard of care treatment (chemo and radiation): 1. "tumor stem cells divide much less often than most cancer cells. Thus, they are less vulnerable to many chemotherapy agents . . . and to radiation"; 2. "data suggests that glioma cells bearing the CD133 biomarker actively resist the effects of chemotherapy and radiation . . . Thus, although standard radiation and chemotherapy treatments kill the proliferating cells that make up most of the tumor, they leave behind, unscathed, a remnant capable of regenerating the deadly mass."

The focus of conventional therapy is wrong and the effort needs to be re-directed. Dr. Foltz told us so. The new researchers are finally starting to think outside the box, using a systems approach to solve the cancer problem, focusing on gene activity, characteristics of cancer stem cells, proteins, and molecular pathways. Why wasn't this shift made years ago, after the failure of chemotherapy was first observed? The basis of the scientific method is a systematic method of observation, experimentation, including trial and error, and the testing of hypotheses. The millions of failed trials by individuals clearly indicate that the toxic method is erroneous. The hypothesis that is the basis for chemotherapy is not proven. The experiment does not compare the results of a treatment group taking chemotherapy against a control group that does not take chemotherapy. The experiment is flawed; the results, as my college statistics professor would say, are "spurious." False, not authentic, not genuine, deceitful. This experiment is a failure, an abysmal failure. It should have been abandoned decades ago, and alternative hypotheses should have been formulated. Yet the cancer industry continued to cling to this hypothesis, regardless of the failure rate. When *will* the establishment come clean? Chemotherapy not only kills healthy cells, but it kills the *wrong cancer cells*. The cancer cells that cause the rapid growth continue to grow unaffected and unchecked by chemotherapy. This is why the oncologists created a "remission" period. They *know* that the cancer will return, and they are waiting for it to return. We are the guinea pigs, participating in a science experiment gone bad. It doesn't work. Dr. Foltz just told us so. Please listen to him.

This is truth. This is the way to wellness.

---

[1]   Dr. Gregory Foltz, "New Hope for Battling Brain Cancer", *Scientific American Mind* Mar/Apr 2010: 50-57.

Tuesday, May18, 2010

41. "Come together . . . right now . . . over me . . ."

Today Jack would have been sixty-one years old. One of the important lessons he taught those of us who loved him was to never pass up an opportunity to celebrate an occasion that required celebrating. I would say that he celebrated every single one of his fifty-two birthdays with a party. Not so much for him, but for us. It was an opportunity for him to gather together everyone he loved in one place. Nothing made him happier. Now, each May 18th is a quiet day. I wait for the party that doesn't happen. I am thankful for all the parties that did.

As birthdays come around seemingly faster and faster each year, many people I know are reluctant to celebrate, or even acknowledge their birthdays. They don't want to be 60 or 57 or 73. We have to realize that birthday celebrations are not for us, they are for the people we love. When people are no longer here to celebrate birthdays, the quietude of that day underscores our loss.

My husband came from a very large family, and the family always celebrated each birthday with gusto: loud, raucous birthday songs punctuated at the end by the clanging of spoons against glasses and plates. The gusto disappeared when the loudest clanger of spoons, my mother-in-law Virginia, died three years ago, on May 17th, her daughter's birthday. Since then, birthday boys and girls have to be coaxed into celebrating. Last year, I wrote an Irish Blessing for my husband, who was bemoaning yet another birthday, and who had to be coaxed into appreciating the life made possible by Virginia.

My Irish Blessing for You
Today make every effort to be happy and celebrate your life.
Be of good cheer!
Accept gracefully gifts and blessings.
Find joy in life.
Appreciate those who love you.
Go for the gusto!

I am grateful to Jack for teaching me how to celebrate my life with the people I love, the people who bring meaning to my life. Birthday celebrations bring people together. Each one is important and should not be allowed to slip past unnoticed. "Life is short," and when you stare death in the face, this trite expression becomes suddenly very real. Enjoy every moment. Don't lose the gusto. The time spent with Jack, especially each May 18th, was a lesson in love: allow others to express their love and accept it with appreciation. Treat others as if they are the most important person in the world. They are.

"Come together . . . right now . . . over me" (The Beatles).

Wednesday, May 26, 2010

42. "In sickness and in health . . ."

May 26, 1984. This is the date of my marriage to my husband Tom, and today is my 26th wedding anniversary. For our silver wedding anniversary, we vacationed in Las Vegas and renewed our wedding vows. This was the happiest day I had experienced in many years. The accumulated grief dissipated like a veil being lifted over a bride's head.

Unexpectedly, I felt as though I was glowing. I felt light, young, happy, almost giddy—very foreign feelings that I had not experienced in years! Strangers approached and asked if we were newly-weds. Everything about the day was perfect. Even being unable to find the correct exit from the hotel casino to walk across the Strip to the Little Chapel of the West was part of the day's adventure. As the time of our vow renewal grew closer, and we were still stuck inside the casino, I remarked to Tom that this was a metaphor for the past twenty-five years: together we were always able to find our way out of any problem or adversity that life brought us. Which way out? We eventually broke free of the darkness of the casino and emerged into the brilliant sunlight. We crossed the street and, once again, professed that we would "love and honor each other, for better or for worse, in sickness and in health, 'til death do us part." We *almost* had one witness, my sister-in-law Sheila, who was delayed due to the presidential limousine closing down the Strip. When we emerged from the chapel, the limousine passed by, and President Obama waved to our little group. We enjoyed a fabulous dinner and anniversary cake on the terrace of the Wynn Hotel, in view of the spectacular waterfall. We stood at the top of *The Hotel at Mandalay Bay* on the outdoor terrace of the Foundation Club viewing the glistening lights of Las Vegas. We ended the evening listening to a live band at the Hard Rock Café. It was a magical day that solidified our commitment to each other and prepared us for the unexpected trials of the upcoming year that started exactly five months later, on October 26th. That was the day of the surgery. That was the day that my husband of twenty-five years leaned over me while I was still recovering, and with tears in his eyes and the determination of steel in his voice, whispered hoarsely, "we *will* grow old together." That was the day that the metaphor became reality, the day that we entered the casino of the oncology world. Which way out? With a lot of luck and perseverance, we broke free of the darkness and emerged into the brilliant sunlight. We found the right way out.

Happy anniversary, honey. My rock. We made it through another year. "For better, for worse." We are both better because of it. "In sickness and in health." We have conquered sickness, and have chosen health. "'Til death do us part." "Do you take this man . . . ?" Yes. I do.

We *will* grow old together. This is our truth: we are each other's inspiration. We are on the way to wellness together. My husband helped me find the truth, and for that, I am forever grateful.

Monday, July 5, 2010

43. Are You Still Alive?

I receive calls from old friends from time to time to see how I am feeling. I jokingly refer to them as the "checking to see if I am still alive calls." I did receive an e-mail from someone, actually asking, "What is going on? Are you still alive?"

I am very much alive, and very much enjoying it! Last night, my husband and I went out with friends on their boat on the Great South Bay to view the Fourth of July fireworks at Fire Island. There is something very calming and reassuring about watching a spectacular firework display while gently being rocked to and fro. We were celebrating the strength and independence not only of our country, but also of the human spirit.

I spent the evening talking to the women, Barbara and Pat, about health issues.

Barbara is an RN, and very much supports and respects my decision. A friend of hers had asked her advice about chemotherapy, and Barbara responded by saying that it is a very personal decision, that her friend should not be scared into making the wrong decision, and that she would have to decide if she can trust her body to heal itself. She told her friend my story, with the hope of bolstering her courage to "just say no to chemo." The friend did go through one round of chemo, and then reported to Barbara that she would "never go through it again, that if she had to feel like that, she would rather be dead." This sentiment was confirmed by Nobel Prize Winner, Charles Huggins, MD, who said, "There are worse things than death. One of them is chemotherapy."[1]

Pat's eighty-seven-year-old father was recently diagnosed with mesothelioma, a disease caused by asbestos exposure that is decreed incurable by the medical establishment. Despite this man's age, and despite the medical belief that this disease is incurable, his doctor recommended chemotherapy. He balked, and Pat told him that he was making the wrong decision. She later reconsidered, thinking that since her father is of sound mind, he has the right to make his own decision. I summarized my cancer odyssey for her, and commended the wisdom of her father's decision, reinforcing her shaky support of his decision. The decision concerning chemo *is* a very personal decision, and it starts with a gut feeling. The fact that I am healthy *because* I refused chemo bolstered her courage to continue to support her father's decision.

There is a bulletin board sponsored by the American Cancer Society, and one of the posts timidly calls out, "Has anyone out there refused chemo?" That person is looking for validation of her own gut feeling. She writes "I am new to this 'nightmare' and I have been told I need chemo. I really, really don't want chemo. I'm worried it will empty our savings account, and I'm not sure I can handle feeling sick for that long. I also can't picture myself without hair. I get the impression nobody ever refuses chemo treatment. I would appreciate any advice. Thanks!" People are looking for answers; they are looking for truth and inspiration to show them the way to wellness.

I am still very much alive, more alive than I have been in years. My hope is that, by sharing these stories, I will reach the people who need this information, and help them discover their own inner courage to "just say no to chemo." Trust your gut; when you do, you will find truth, you will find inspiration, and you will discover the way to wellness.

---

[1]   *Healing Cancer from the Inside Out*, dir. Mike Anderson, DVD, 2008).

Sunday, July 11, 2010

44. On the Right Path

There are encouraging signs that the researchers are finally getting it right. There is a glimmer of hope. Big Pharma has finally discovered that the key to health is the immune system, after holding stubbornly and steadfastly to the "search and destroy" strategy it deployed for over forty (40) years. The mission has been to destroy the tumor. If the patient dies in the process, well at least the tumor has been destroyed. The industry has finally learned that the key to disrupting the momentum of the disease is through the immune system.

◊   A recent news article[1] reported that the FDA approved a new treatment for prostate cancer that activates the immune system to fight the disease. This is a novel approach for corporate medicine, but it is not novel for the alternative medicines. Alternative medicines have been using, or trying to use this approach for years, often thwarted by the interventions of the FDA. Dendreon Corporation's Provenge is the first immunotherapy drug to receive the approval of the FDA. Dendreon's stock dropped three (3) years ago after the FDA withheld approval for this treatment, despite an expert panel's recommendation for approval. The "little 'Pharma' that could" persevered and successfully brought an efficacious treatment to market, despite the FDA hurdle. During this three (3) year delay, thousands of lives could have been saved.

According to the article, the side effects of Provenge are mild in comparison to the side effects of chemotherapy, which include "hair loss, nausea, anemia and diarrhea." The article neglects to mention all the other devastating side effects of chemotherapy, which include healthy cell, immune system destruction, organ destruction, neuropathy, and potentially death.

The article further reports, "Currently doctors treat cancer by surgically removing tumors, attacking them with chemotherapy drugs or blasting them with radiation. Provenge offers an important fourth approach by directing the body's natural defense mechanisms against the disease." Medical specialists stressed that it is "an addition to current medical practice, not a replacement," with one practitioner stating, "This is just one step in a new pathway for treating patients."

Reporting on that same breakthrough, *The New York Times* states, "The broader strategy uses a drug that could potentially become a universal treatment for all types of cancer. It works by releasing a brake on the body's immune system, letting the immune system attack the cancer more vigorously."[2]

The face-saving spin by corporate medicine is to present this as yet another weapon in the arsenal in the war against cancer; the generals will not admit that the original battle plan was wrong. But at least now they are seemingly allowing the emergence of the right plan, the *only* plan that can lead the way to good health.

◊ At the annual conference of the American Society of Clinical Oncology in Chicago, progress was revealed in the treatment of melanoma. A Little Pharma (Medarex, Inc) researched a drug that helps the immune system fight tumors.

This company was bought out by Big Pharma (Bristol-Myers) which is trying to push the drug Ipilimumab through the hurdles of the FDA. Researchers ambitiously believe that the drug could be available by the end of 2010. In the meantime, 50,000 people die annually, worldwide. The American Cancer Society admits, "We're asking questions that should have been answered decades ago."[3,4]

◊ In findings presented at the same annual meeting of the American Society of Clinical Oncology, a Mayo clinic study shows potential for the use of epigallocatechin gallate (EGCG), the major component of green tea, in reducing cancer cells in chronic lymphocytic leukemia (CLL) patients. "These studies advance the notion that a nutraceutical like EGCG can and should be studied as cancer preventives," says Neil Kay, MD, a hematology researcher whose laboratory first tested the green tea extract in leukemic blood cells from CLL patients. "Using non-toxic chemicals to push back cancer growth to delay the need for toxic therapies is a worthy goal in oncology research . . ."[5] If we have to refer to naturally occurring substances such as EGCG in green tea as "nutra*ceuticals*" in order for these substances to be recognized as treatment options, then this is a concession that we need to make so that corporate medicine can save face and allow these non-toxic options to be presented by the medical community to cancer patients.

◊ In a video presented by Dr. William Li (President and Medical Director of the Angiogenesis Foundation) "Can we starve cancer?," Dr. Li discusses anti-angiogenesis, which blocks the growth of blood vessels that feed a tumor.[6] Blood vessels grow during certain times and in certain situations. During a period of disease, the body's regulation of blood vessel growth goes awry; too many blood vessels in the body can feed a cancerous disease. The body's anti-angiogenesis is out of balance: this is "a hallmark of every type of cancer." Cancer cells can't grow without a blood supply. By cutting off the blood supply, anti-angiogenesis is achieved, and the cancers can't become dangerous. Dr. Li refers to this as "cancer without disease." Anti-angiogenesis is the "tipping point" between harmless and harmful cancers. It differs from chemotherapy in that it selectively aims at the blood vessels that are feeding cancer. Since 2004, when this type of therapy became available, Dr. Li notes that there was a 70%-100% improvement in certain types of cancers, but he questioned, "why not an improvement in *all* cancers?" He reasoned that since diet causes approximately one-third of all environmentally caused cancers, why not *eat to starve cancer*? The known superfoods (parsley, garlic, red grapes, berries, teas, cooked tomatoes) are all anti-angiogenesis agents. Consumption of these foods is key to keeping cancer at bay, by starving cancer to death.

There is hope that finally some researchers are brave enough to break away from the pack, away from the "preponderance of medical opinion," and are exploring new pathways to help lead us back to wellness. In finding the truth, there is inspiration.

---

[1] Matthew Perrone, "FDA approves breakthrough cancer therapy Provenge," *Associated Press*, 29 Apr 2010.

[2] Andrew Pollack, "Scientists Cite Advances on Two Kinds of Cancer," *The New York Times*, 5 Jun 2010.

[3] Marilynn Marchione, "Drug boosts survival in major skin cancer study," *Associated Press*, 5 Jun 2010.

[4] Marilynn Marchione, "Cancer wins may be bigger than they seem," *Associated Press*, 9 Jun 2010.

[5] Karl Oestreich, "Green tea extract appears to keep cancer in check in majority of CLL patients," <http://newsblog.mayoclinic.org/2010/06/04/green-tea-extract-appears-to-keep-cancer-in-check-in-majority-of-cll-patients/>.

[6] *Can we starve cancer?*, Dr. William Li, <<http://www.ted.com/talks/ william_ li.html>>, 2010.

Sunday, July 11, 2010

45. Lemmings

Lemmings are characterized as strange creatures that commit mass suicide for no apparent reason. This is an unsubstantiated myth, and may actually be an accident of nature which occurs during migration, rather than an intentional act. Lemmings do swim, and they may actually be attempting to cross a body of water, albeit unsuccessfully, in search of a better place.

The myth is the basis for the video game *Lemmings*, in which the player must stop the lemmings from mindlessly marching over cliffs. Because of their association with this self-destructive behavior, lemming suicide has made its way into the vernacular to describe "people who go along unquestioningly with popular opinion, with potentially dangerous or fatal consequences."[1]

Like the lemmings, mainstream cancer patients are following the wrong path that has been set by corporate medicine. With the unwitting support of family and friends, and popular opinion, they are mindlessly marching off cliffs or bravely navigating dangerous waters, and suffering dangerous or fatal consequences, while believing that they are migrating to a better place. These cancer patients are not intentionally committing suicide; if they were, they would have engaged Dr. Kevorkian. They are unintentionally dying, by willingly agreeing to submit to "maximum sub-lethal doses of chemotherapy." We need to ferret out the truth.

It has long been accepted that lemmings are suicidal; they may just be unlucky, or uninformed, or they may just be unaware of the impact of their choices. It has also been long accepted that chemo is the acceptable treatment for cancer, and that people die of *cancer*. This is not truth. Chemo does not help. *People die of chemo, not of cancer.* Cancer is a manageable disease. Find the truth.

The cancer industry has triggered the stampede of the lemmings, and is standing by, counting their money, watching everyone charge off the cliff to certain death. We need to stop, get our bearings, and find our own sense of direction back to safety. We need to follow someone who can lead us away from the edge of the cliff and back on the path to excellent health. We need truth and inspiration.

---

[1]   Wikipedia, <http://www.wikipedia.org>.

Sunday, July 11, 2010

46. Better Living—NOT through Chemistry

For over seventy years, the E. I. du Pont de Nemours and Company has espoused their corporate slogan "Better Things for Better Living Through Chemistry."[1,2] But has living become better with chemistry? The documentary *Gasland* is about the insidious incursion of natural gas companies into over thirty (30) states to engage in a process referred to as "hydraulic fracturing" or "fracking" in order to mine natural gas.[3] This process drills 8,000 feet underground and injects over 596 chemicals, many of them known carcinogens. Animals are dying, people are sick, tap water catches fire. Halliburton is one of the major players. These small sites are exempt from all the environmental laws, thanks to our former leaders, Cheney and Bush who pushed through the 2005 Energy Bill, commonly referred to as the "Halliburton Loophole."[4] Caveat emptor: be careful when you buy a property; if fracking has occurred upstream, your water supply may be contaminated. These companies go in and pay people off for rights to drill on their properties; they do not disclose the potential health hazards, they deny that the water is unsafe, and the only recourse is to take corporate America to court. The individual homeowner is in a David and Goliath scenario. The environmental protection agencies are useless when it comes to protecting the environment against fracking, but very useful in supporting on-land drilling for natural oil. According to one Environmental Protection Agency (EPA) official, the EPA is "asleep at the wheel." Speaking about the industry leaders, Congressman Maurice Hinchey stated that people were not being honest about what they were doing, they were finding the least expensive way to get the highest profits.[5] The current administration calls these wells "safe," despite evidence to the contrary. Start with the truth; the truth is not optional.

The natural gas corporations, like the pharmaceutical corporations, have created a systematic culture of non-disclosure of material facts. They are hiding behind the "corporate veil." Consumers are in harm's way, in a situation created by corporate greed. The public is *not* told the truth. The "corporate veil" must be pierced and the truth must be revealed.

How can this happen in America? We are sickened by chemicals, and then chemicals are used to treat the chemically-caused diseases, and the chemical treatments for the chemically-caused diseases make us sicker, not better. Abandon DuPont's corporate slogan: chemistry is *not* the answer for better living. It is *not* the truth. It is *not* the way to wellness.

[1] Dr. John Kenly Smith, "DuPont: The Enlightened Organization," <http://www2.dupont.com/Heritage/en_US/Enlightened/Enlightened.html>.

[2] Wikipedia, <http://en.Wikipedia.org/wiki/chemotherapy>.

[3] *Gasland*, Dir. Josh Fox, International WOW Company, Documentary, 2010.

[4] Alison Rose Levy, "Gasland: Will New York become the next casualty of the Halliburton Loophole?", <http://www.huffingtonpost.com/alison-rose-levy/gasland-will-new-york-be_b_617072.html>.

[5] *Gasland*, op. cit.

Saturday, July 17, 2010

47. The Hummingbird

   This morning, as I completed this labor of love, a rare hummingbird appeared outside my window, drawing nectar from the purple petunias. These flowers have a special significance: my friend Taylor gave me a hanging planter of purple petunias on one of our last visits. Every year since her death, I buy a planter of purple petunias. When I look at these flowers, I am looking at Taylor.

   Curious about the sudden appearance of this rare creature, I googled "hummingbird" and found the following, a fitting ending to these stories:

   "Hummingbird's Teachings Include:

   Hummingbird darts from flower to flower in search of nectar and teaches all who honor her to let in the beauty of life, the nectar of love. This tiny bird is surprisingly tough and aggressive, often driving away larger birds. Invoke Hummingbird for indomitable energy and the ability to tap great power from within.

   What is hummingbird's message for us? First of all, adaptability in life's many situations and being able to roll with the punches.

   Hummingbird is a very good sign. She is a good-luck messenger. She takes our prayers to the Great Creator. She is a doctor and healer. The Hummingbird has the power to travel long distances under great odds and obstacles. Hummingbird's Wisdom Includes:

> *Accomplishing All Against Impossible Odds*
> *Finding Good in People*
> *Being Adaptable in Life's Many Situations*
> *Spreading Joy and Love to All*
> *Searching for the Sweetness of Life*
> *Inner Joy*
> *Finding Unique Ways to Awaken Others to Beauty*
> *Energetically Tasting the Sweetness of Life*
> *Clarity*
> *Lucidity*
> *Optimism*
> *Stopping Time*
> *Having a Warrior Spirit*
> *Being Feisty*
> *Agility*
> *Transcending Time*

Hummingbird Empowerment: Animals have gifts that they are willing to offer people. One gift of the animals is their energies to empower people on their journey of life. With their energy gift, each animal offers their particular wisdom to the person. For people who need to fill their lives with wonder, Hummingbird offers his formidable gifts." [1]

Find your truth and inspiration every day. It is right outside your window. It will come to you like the hummingbird. Recognize the meaning of it, and understand the message it brings. Become the hummingbird. Internalize every quality of this creature: strength, joy, love, energy, power. This is your way to wellness. Trust it, and only then, in the words of Jerry Garcia, *"We WILL survive."* (Touch of Gray).

The writing of these stories became part of my healing process, healing body, mind, spirit, psyche. It became my mission in life to expose the pharmaceutical companies for the role that they continue to play in the stagnation of beneficial cancer treatments. Through these stories, I have articulated my outrage and disappointment at the failure of the oncological medical establishment to adequately address this disease; my hope is to help and inspire other people to choose the right path. These stories are greater than a chronicling of one person's odyssey through the cancer labyrinth, greater than an exposé of the cancer industry. The *individual* stories chronicle my discovery of both truth and inspiration on the way to wellness. But the *collective* stories are the gestalt of my cancer odyssey. They are meant to provoke thought about what we as a nation are doing to ourselves to make us all so unhealthy: chemically-infused, prepared foods; chemically-infused, toxic environmental conditions; and chemically-derived medications for cancer and for every other imagined and imaginable ailment and disease. Corporate America—corporate gas, corporate food, corporate drugs, corporate cancer treatment—is killing Americans to feed their corporate greed.

The answer is in non-toxic treatments—natural treatments which are beneficial to the body. Abandon the mustard gas approach to treating disease. Embrace the alternative methods. Just say no to chemo.

This is truth. This is inspiration. This is the way to wellness.

And now I am going for a run . . . I am on my way to wellness.

---

[1]   "Animal Teachers Winged Ones." <http://www.funkman.org/animal/ bird/ hummingbird.html>.

~~~

Wednesday, August 18, 2010

48. Afterword

Today is my birthday. Ten (10) months ago, I feared that I would not live to see this day. This past year has been an odyssey for which I am grateful. I have survived a dreaded disease, and have done so *because* I did not choose the toxic chemicals of chemotherapy. I am robustly healthy. When I first told family, friends, neighbors, and co-workers that I declined "conventional" treatment, most of them looked at me in amazement and tried to convince me to go along with the program. Now, they eye me guardedly, ask how I am feeling, tell me that I look wonderful, and then acknowledge that I must be "on to something."

My "incredible journey" would not have been possible without the help, love, care, and concern of my husband, family, friends, neighbors, co-workers, and team of alternative health care practitioners, and I thank them and acknowledge all with love.

Somehow I was inspired to journalize my odyssey. My birthday wish is that others will be drawn to my message, and that they will recognize the truth and be inspired to start out on their own "way to wellness." It is my birthday wish, that in my lifetime, before all my birthdays are past, that chemotherapy will be exposed for the fraud that it is.

Understand that the cancer business really *is* about the money. The American Cancer Society (ACS) reports that cancer is the world's top "economic killer," at the worldwide cost of almost $900 billion in 2008, in terms of productivity and lost life. The ACS states that the amount of money devoted to cancer "is way out of whack with the impact it has [on the economy]." The UN General Assembly called for a meeting to examine this issue, which is being compared to "the global initiative that led to big increases in spending on AIDS."[1] Understand that the ACS is a shill for Big Pharma.[2] Understand that the focus of the "War on Cancer" is to bring more money into the system, and *not* to find a cure for the disease. Understand that the focus of this new "global initiative" will be on the *money*, and *not* on the *cure*. Once you understand this, your decision to choose a beneficial, alternative treatment will be easy.

Today, as I am letting this book go, I am also letting the experience of cancer go. The storm is behind me. Sunny skies are ahead.

> "They say it's your birthday . . .
> We're gonna have a good time . . .
> I'm glad it's your birthday . . .
> Happy Birthday to you . . .
> I would like you to dance . . .
> Take a cha cha cha chance . . ." (The Beatles).

---

[1] Marilynn Marchione, "Cancer's high toll on world's economy," *Newsday*, 17 Aug 2010.

[2] *Healing Cancer from the Inside Out*, dir. Mike Anderson, DVD, 2008).

Saturday, January 29, 2011

49. The Last Word . . . .

I am doing a final review of this manuscript, and drinking a cup of "Supreme Quality Green Tea" from Rwanda, the only tea in the world actually (reportedly) *imported* by China. We know that green tea contains polyphenols, which are anticancer agents. What is interesting about this particular tea is that the packaging states "Believed to inhibit an enzyme responsible for cancer cell growth and said to kill cultured cancer cells with no ill-effect on healthy cells." This is a claim that could *not* be made by a green tea imported into the U.S.

My neighbor Bridget's daughter is undergoing treatment in Germany, almost three (3) years after a renowned cancer center told her she had six (6) months to live and to go home and have a sirloin steak and an ice cream sundae. Today Bridget brought me a website page from Epeius Biotechnologies.[1] In Greek mythology, Epeius was the designer of the original Trojan Horse, and Epeius Biotechnologies has developed a "tumor-targeted delivery vehicle,"—a "Trojan Horse . . ." This is the future of cancer treatments. The new biotech companies are thinking outside of the box, recognizing that the "standard of care" chemotherapy treatments do not work. Mainstream "Big Pharma" is on the wrong track, which is why Bridget's daughter and others still have to leave the country for beneficial medical care. We need an Epeius, a Trojan Horse, to win the battle against Big Pharma. Twenty-five years ago, Mary Yevchak had to leave the country for beneficial medical care. In the words of the Beatles, "Nothing's gonna change my world." Things have not changed much in a quarter of a century in our American world, and things will *not* change unless we demand change. American citizens should not have to leave this country in the year 2011 to obtain the medical treatment of their choice. Companies should be permitted to import healthy products and to honestly describe what the beneficial effects of those products are, without censure. Demand change. Demand truth. Be inspired by Rwandan green tea. Be inspired by the efforts of Mary Yevchak and Bridget's daughter, and all others who are fighting, not only cancer, but the larger battle against the cancer industry. Be part of the thought revolution. This is truth. This is inspiration.

---

[1]   Epeius Biotechnologies. <http://www.epeiusbiotech.com>.

Bibliography

Websites:

"20 Health Benefits of Turmeric." <http://www.healthdiaries.com/eatthis/20-health-benefits-of-turmeric.html>.

"Alkaline Foods / Acidic Foods." <http://wwwctds.info/acidic-foods.html>.

"American Medical Association." <http://www.encognitive.com/node/1209>.

"Animal Teachers Winged Ones." <http://www.funkman.org/animal/ bird/ hummingbird.html>.

"Apricot Seeds Kill Cancer Cells without Side Effects." <http://www. naturalnews.com/027088_cancer_laetrile_health.html>.

"Are We Treating Cancer but Killing the Patient?" Dr. George J Georgiou, Ph.D.,ND.,D.Sc (AM), <http://www.rawfoodinfo.com/articles/art_ Arewetreatingcancerbutkillingpatient.htm>.

"B 17, Vitamin B17—Amygdalin, Almond, B17—Laetrile, Improve Immune System with B17." <http://www.dreambandclub.com/health_free_ articles_B17.htm>.

"B17 (Laetrile) & Nutrition in the Treatment of Cancer." "http://www. curesnaturally.com/Articles/Cancer/Cancer56.html>.

"Because you need the right info to make the right decision." <http://www. ChemoFraud.com>.

"Can You Trust Chemotherapy to Cure Your Cancer?" <http://www.natural news.com/023689_chemotherapy_cancer_disease.html>.

"Cancer Facts & Figures 2010." American Cancer Society. 2010. <http://www.cancer.org/Research/CancerFactsFigures/CancerFactsFigures/cancer-facts-and-figures-2010>.

"Cancer Surgery Special Report—Life Extension." < http://www.lef.org/featured-articles/Cancer-Surgery-Special-Report.htm>.

"Cancer Update E-mail—It's a Hoax!" <http://www.hopkinsmedicine.org/kimmel_cancer_center/news_events/featured/cancer_update_e-mail_it_is_a_hoax.html>.

"Cancerolytic Herbs: a History of Suppression." <http://health.centreforce.com/health/industry.html>.

"Chemotherapy: Does It Really Cause Cancer?"<http://searchwarp.com/swa78335.htm>.

"Chiropractic History—AMA v. Chiropractic." <http://www.svpvril.com/amavchir.html>.

"DeGette, Polis introduce FRAC Act aimed at closing hydraulic fracturing 'loophole'."<http://degette.house.gov/index.php?option=com_content&view=article&id=773:degette-polis-introduce-frac-act-aimed-at-closing-hydraulic-fracturing-loophole&catid=66:in-the-news&Itemid=195>.

Daenell ND, Carrie Louise. "Resveratrol on 60 Minutes." <http://www.selfgrowthcom/articles/Resveratrol_on_60_Minutes.html>.

Epeius Biotechnologies. <http://www.epeiusbiotech.com>.

"Exposing the FRAUD behind the Chemotherapy Industry." <http://www.chemofraud.com>.

"FDA: 187 Fake Cancer "Cures" Consumers Should Avoid." <http://www.fda.gov/Drugs/GuidanceComplianceRegulatoryInformation/EnforcementActivitiesbyFDA/ucm171057.htm>.

"FDA (Food and Drug Administration) War Against Cancer Cure!" <http://www.apfn.org/thewinds/1997/09/bruce_halstead.html>.

"FDA Warns of Internet Sales of Fake Cancer Cures." <http://www.healthnews.com/alerts-outbreaks/fda-warns-against-internet-sales-fake-cancer-cures-1257.html>.

"Fraud: Chemotherapy." <http://www.mnwelldir.org/docs/fraud/chemo.htm>.

"Gerson Institute Healing with Nature." <http://gerson.org/Programs/findgersonclinic.htm>.

"Guolin Qi Gong-Cancer Buster. Walking Qi Gong." <http://www.qigongchinesehealth.com/walking_qigong>.

"Heal Cancer NATURALLY | NO chemotherapy | NO Radiation or Surgery." <http://www.cancer-free-for-life.com>.

"How Chi Gong Works on Cancer," <http://wwwhealthy foundations.com/guolin/guolin_article.html>.

"| Illuminati News | Chemo A FRAUD—More Evidence It's WORTHLESS." <http://www.illuminati-news.com/Articles/113.html>.

"In-Hospital Deaths from Medical Errors at 195,000 per year, HealthGrades Study Finds." <http://www.healthgrades.com/media/DMS/pdf/InhosptialDeathsPatientSafetyPressRelease072704.pdf. [sic].

James, David. "A Last Stand, An American Tragedy. Testimony of Mary and Michael Yevchak, Congressional Public Hearing." <http://www.cancercontrolinfo.com/ index2B.html>.

"Jason Vale and the Cancer Mafia," <http://www.apricotsfromgod.info/ jvale/>.

Lerner, Michael. "Choices In Healing: Integrating the Best of Conventional and Complementary Approaches to Cancer." <http://www.commonweal.org/ pubs/choices/4.html>.

Levy, Alison Rose. "Gasland: Will New York become the next casualty of the Halliburton Loophole?" <http://www.huffingtonpost.com/alison-rose-levy/gasland-will-new-york-be_b_617072.html>.

Life Extension Foundation. <http://www.lef.org>.

"List of Alkaline Foods | Acid Alkaline Food." <http://www.energiseforlife. com/list_of_alkaline_foods.php>.

"Lothar Hirneise's Book Chemotherapy Heals Cancer and the World is Flat: Extract/Table of Contents." <http://www.healingcancernaturally.com/ hirneise-chemotherapy-cures.html>.

"Louise Hay | Author and Founder of Hay House, Inc." <http://www.louisehay. com/affirmations/index.php>.

"Lovaza."<http://www.lovaza.com>.

Marchione, Marilynn. "Cancer wins may be bigger than they seem." June 9, 2010. <http://www.washingtonpost.com/wp-dyn/content/article /2010/06/09/ AR2010060903747_pf.html>.

Marchione, Marilynn. "Drug boosts survival in major skin cancer study." June 5, 2010. <http://www.newsday.com/business/drug-boosts-survival- in-major—skin-cancer-study-1.1983769>.

"Memorable Quotes for 'Network'." <http://www.imdb.com/title/tt0074958/ quotes>.

"Memorial Sloan-Kettering Cancer Center."<http://www.mskcc.org/ mskcc/ html/511.cfm>.

Moss, Ph.D., Ralph W. "Cancer Decisions." <http://www.cancerdecisions. com>.

"National Cancer Institute a 'rudderless ship'."<http://www.psa-rising.com/ blog/2009/08/national-cancer-institute-a-rudderless-ship/>.

"National Cancer Institute Factsheet" <http://www.cancer.gov/cancertopics/ factsheet/Therapy/tamoxifen>.

"National Health Freedom Action." <http://www.nationalhealthfreedom. org/>.

"Natural Remedies, Natural Health, Natural Cures, Herbal Remedies, Natural Medicine." <http://www.naturalcures.com>.

"New Cancer Treatments—Independent Cancer Research Foundation, Inc." <http://www.new-cancer-treatments.org>.

"Nutritional Health Balancing Program. Artificial Sweeteners." <http://www.pacifichealthcenter.com/blog/71-artificial-sweeteners/>.

Oestreich, Karl. "Green tea extract appears to keep cancer in check in majority of CLL patients." June 4, 2010. <http://newsblog.mayoclinic.org/2010/06/04/ green-tea-extract-appears-to-keep-cancer-in-check-in-majority-of-cll-patients/>.

"Oncologists profit on chemotherapy drugs they prescribe to cancer patients." Apr. 2006. <http://www.mesothel.com/asbestos-cancer/mesothelioma/chemotherapy/alimta/alimta_profit.htm>.

Pollack, Andrew. "Scientists Cite Advances on Two Kinds of Cancer." June 5, 2010. <http://www.nytimes.com/2010/06/06/health/research/ 06cancer.html? sq=melanoma&st=cse&scp=1&pagewanted=print>.

"Ralph Moss on Cancer—Expert Guidance for Crucial Decision." <http://www.ralphmoss.com/html/naessens1.shtml>.

"Redwood Caregiver Resource Center."<http://www.redwoodcrc.org/fact Sheets/Parkinsons/XGlossaryOfTerms.doc>.

Reimer, Helena. "The Gerson Institute." <http://www.ezinearticles.com/? The-Gerson-Institute&id=3494956>.

Ross, Ph. D., R. and Pelton, Lee Overholser. "ALTERNATIVES IN CANCER THERAPY." <http://www.curezone.com/diseases/cancer/laetrile.asp>.

Scholberg, Andrew. "Reagan's cancer treated in Germany." <http:// freegrab.net/Reagan%27s%20cancer%20treated%20in%20Germany.htm >.

Smith, Dr. John Kenly. "DuPont: The Enlightened Organization." <http://www2.dupont.com/Heritage/en_US/Enlightened/Enlightened.html>.

"Stop High Fructose Corn Syrup! HFCS free foods." <http://www.stophfcs.com/list.html>.

"TED Talks. William Li: Can we eat to starve cancer?" <http //www.ted.com/talks/william_li.html>.

"The Danger in Drug Kickbacks." The New York Times. 14 May 2007. <http://www.nytimes.com/2007/05/14/opinion/14mon1.html?_r=1>.

"The Dirty Little Secret between the FDA and Drug Industry—Share the Wealth." <http://www.communicationagents.com/chris/2004/08/26/the_dirty_little_secret_between_the_fda_and_drug_industry.htm>.

"The saliva PH test and cancer." <http://wwwhealingdaily.com/conditions/saliva-ph-test.htm>.

"The War between Orthodox Medicine and Alternative Medicine." <http://www.cancertutor.com>.

"Vitamin B17 and Laetrile in Australia." <http://www.laetrile.com.au>.

"Vitamin B-17—Laetrile—Anti-cancer Properties." <http://www.healingdaily.com/detoxification-diet/vitamin-b-17-laetrile.htm>.

"Walking Qigong (Guolin Qigong)—The Anti-Cancer Qigong." <http://www.qigongchinesehealth.com/walking_qigong>.

"Ways to strengthen the immune system." <http://www.essortment.com/all/immunesystemst_rzzb.htm>.

"Why Alternative Cancer Treatment Chemotherapy in Oncology." <http://www.healingcancernaturally.com/chemotherapy-cancer-treatment.html>.

Wikipedia. <http://www.wikipedia.org>.

Wilson, Duff. "Harvard Teaching Hospitals Cap Outside Pay" The New York Times. 2 Jan. 2010. <http://www.nytimes.com/2010/01/03/health/research/03hospital.html?emc=eta1>.

Wilson, Duff. "Harvard Medical School in Ethics Quandary." The New York Times. 2 Mar. 2009. <http://www.nytimes.com/2009/03/03/business/03medschool.html?emc=eta1</div>.

Articles:

Faloon, William. "So Many Needless Cancer Deaths." *Life Extension* December 2009: 7-12.

Foltz, Dr. Gregory. "New Hope for Battling Brain Cancer." *Scientific American Mind* March/April 2010: 50-57.

Marchione, Marilynn. "Cancer's high toll on world's economy." *Newsday* August 17, 2010.

Perrone, Matthew. "FDA approves breakthrough cancer therapy Provenge." *Newsday* April 29, 2010.

CDs and DVDs:

Australia. Dir. Baz Luhrmann. DVD. Bazmark Films, 2008.

Cancer: Discovering your Healing Power. Dir. Louise Hay. DVD. Hay House, Inc., 2004.

Caroline Myss' Chakra Meditation Music. Music by Stevin McNamara. CD. Sound True. 2002.

Food, Inc. Dir. Robert Kenner. DVD. Documentary, 2008.

Gasland. Dir. Josh Fox, International WOW Company, Documentary, 2010.

Healing Cancer from the Inside Out. Dir. Mike Anderson. DVD. Documentary, 2008.

Our Exclusive Guo Lin Chi Gong Video. <http://www.healthyfoundations.com/guolin/guolinvideo.html>.

Qigong Beginning Practice with Francesco Garripoli & Daisy Lee-Garripoli. Dir. Michael Badertscher. DVD. Gaiam, Inc., 2004.

Songs of Kuan Yin. CD. Sounds True, 2008.

The Beautiful Truth. Dir. Steve Kroschel. DVD. Documentary, 2008.

The Law of Attraction. Dir Esther and Jerry Hicks. CD. Hay House, Inc., 2007.

Books:

Campbell Douglass II, William. *Hydrogen Peroxide: Medical Miracle*. Panama: Rhino Publishing, SA, 2003.

Cavanaugh, Madison. *The One-Minute Cure: The Secret to Healing Virtually all Diseases*. Beverly Hills: Think-Outside-the-Book Publishing, Inc., 2008.

Greer, MD, MPH, Julia. *The Anti-Cancer Cookbook*. North Branch, MN: Sunrise River Press, 2008.

Hay, Louise L. *You Can Heal Your Life*. New York: Hay House, 2008.

Irving, John. *Last Night in Twisted River*. New York: Random House, 2009.

Life Extension Foundation. *FDA: Failure, Deception, Abuse: The Story of an Out-of-Control Government Agency and What it Means for your Health*. Mount Jackson, VA: Praktikos Books, 2010.

Lynes, Barry. *The Healing of Cancer, The Cures-The Cover-ups and the Solution Now!* Ontario, Canada: Marcus Books, 1989.

McCabe, Ed. *Flood Your Body with Oxygen*. Carson City, NV: Energy Publications, LLC, 2008.

McKeith, Dr. Gillian. *Living Food for Health: 12 Natural Superfoods to Transform your Health*. London: Piatkus Books, 2000.

Myss, PhD, Caroline. *Anatomy of the Spirit: The Seven Stages of Power and Healing*. New York: Three Rivers Press, Crown Publishing Group, a division of Random House, Inc., 1996.

Null, PhD, Gary. *Death by Medicine*. Mount Jackson, VA: Praktikos Books, 2010.

Quillen, PhD, Patrick. *Beating Cancer with Nutrition*. Carlsbad, CA: Nutrition Times Press, Inc., 2005.

Simon, MD, David. *Return to Wholeness: Embracing Body, Mind, and Spirit in the Face of Cancer*. New York: John Wiley & Sons, Inc., 1999.

Somers, Suzanne. *Knockout: Interviews with Doctors who are Curing Cancer and How to Prevent Getting it in the First Place*. New York: Crown Publishing Group, a division of Random House, Inc., 2009.

Any omission is unintentional.